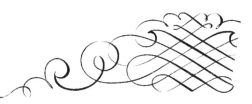

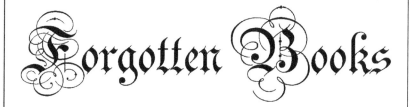
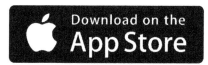
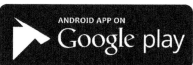

ISBN 978-1-332-27069-9
PIBN 10307098

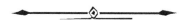

MORBID CRAVING FOR MORPHIA.

(*DIE MORPHIUMSUCHT.*)

A MONOGRAPH FOUNDED ON PERSONAL OBSERVATIONS.

BY

EDWARD LEVINSTEIN, M.D.

MEDICAL DIRECTOR OF THE MAISON DE SANTÉ:
SCHÖNEBERG-BERLIN.

TRANSLATED FROM THE GERMAN
BY
CHARLES HARRER, M.D., L.R.C.P. LOND.

PHYSICIAN TO THE EASTERN DISPENSARY OF THE
GERMAN HOSPITAL IN LONDON.

LONDON:
SMITH, ELDER, & CO., 15 WATERLOO PLACE.
1878.

PREFACE.

———◆◦◆———

IT is not my intention in this work to write on the importance of Morphia from the time of its first introduction into the treatment of diseases. I must likewise abstain from mentioning the reasons which prevented Germany from enjoying the benefits of the method of subcutaneous injections of morphia for a period of six years after its first introduction into England by Wood, and its extensive use in France.

The scope of this work is limited, its sole object being to clearly demonstrate the ill effects which continued injections of morphia have upon the human body; to show the dangers threatening society by such a continuous use of the drug; and to point out the remedies for the redress of this abuse.

THE AUTHOR.

SCHÖNEBERG-BERLIN :
January, 1877.

CONTENTS.

MORBID CRAVING FOR MORPHIA.

THE subcutaneous injection of morphia has, until the last few years, been but rarely practised in Germany. The facility of Pravaz's method, however, its rapid and marvellous action in relieving pain, and the calming effect it had upon the sick and wounded during the war of 1866, paved the way for its adoption in this country. The scope of its application was extended daily without the slightest discrimination, and very soon this narcotic remedy was used to remove every abnormal sensation, whether caused by neuropathic or inflammatory action ; consequently the rational treatment became endangered by the modern method. The patients appeared to be doing well under their morphia intoxication; but at the same time the prominent features of the disease, *i.e.* the diagnosis, gradually became obscure. The most prominent scientific men foresaw the danger which would result from this mania for morphia injections; and by the bedside of the patient, as well as at the

B

teacher's desk, spoke earnestly against its use, but without avail.

The enthusiasm of the general public for this remedy, on account of its marvellous action, spread rapidly; and finding out that injections of morphia also relieved physical pain, they soon took out of the hands of the medical man a remedy which, when only in the latter's possession, would have remained a blessing for suffering humanity.

Here begins the history of the disease I am going to describe, and to which I have given the name of 'morbid craving for morphia.' The correctness of the name might be called in question, others having proposed to call it Morphinismus, Morphia-delirium, and Morphia-evil. Neither of these three designations sufficiently answer to the character of the disease as delineated by me. A patient who has for some months been treated with injections of morphia, on account of an acute and painful disease, may show all the symptoms of Morphinismus, *i.e.* of specific morphia poisoning; but if, on the termination of his illness, he does not feel any desire for more of the drug, he has no 'morbid craving for morphia.' On the other hand, an individual may for years have a craving for morphia without showing the least symptoms of Morphinismus. For this very reason, the name of Morphia-evil will be unacceptable, and still less the name of Morphio-mania, unless we desire to characterise the morbid craving for morphia as due to a diseased state of the mind :

but the latter is only one of the symptoms which, when the drug is withheld, may or may not appear without in the least altering the character of the case.

Morbid craving for morphia means the uncontrollable desire of a person to use morphia as a stimulant and tonic, and the diseased state of the system caused by the injudicious use of the said remedy.

Under this head we do not include those cases which necessitate the use of morphia for special medical purposes. Its proper use in these cases prevents the patient getting accustomed to the drug, because the injections are discontinued as soon as the disease passes away. But this can only be decided by the medical man, who has himself administered the injections, and never by the patient, if perchance they have been left in his hands. All painful diseases accompanied with sleeplessness make the convalescents nervous and melancholy; they continually worry themselves about their bodily health, greatly magnifying the importance of every trifling bodily change, of which a healthy person would not have taken the slightest notice. If, then, they should have by them a remedy, such as injection of morphia, which has previously proved of great benefit to them, they will at once resort to its use, either to prevent pain coming on, or to avoid the recurrence of a restless night. Such are the causes of the habitual use of morphia, of the seeming impossibility of doing without it, and, finally, the morbid craving for it.

The originators and propagators of this disease
are the medical men who, in cases more or less
painful and protracted, have advised the patients
to themselves use the injection of morphia. They
must not be blamed for acting as they did, as it was
done in the hope of affording relief to their patients,
none of them thinking of the attendant danger. The
evil was still further spread by those suffering from
craving for morphia, who highly praised it as a
remedy of which they knew the beneficial effects.

The injections of morphia not only relieve sleeplessness and pain, but their action at the same time
induces a change in the entire system. It produces
a state of mental excitement that can only be compared to that produced by the use of alcohol. The
temper is altered ; depressed persons will become
lively ; to the fainting person it imparts strength ; to
the weakly it restores energy ; the taciturn become
eloquent ; shy persons lose their bashfulness ; and
the consciousness of power and ability is greatly increased. But as soon as the morphia has left the
system, a reaction sets in, and the period of great
mental and bodily excitement is followed by a state
of deep despondency.

This narcotic remedy will soon be indispensable
to those who have it often injected, as, by doing so,
they know that they are able to banish all physical
and moral trouble ; hence they resort to morphia as
the drunkard to the dram bottle. They drown their
anger, their domestic sorrows, and their business

cares; and, like the drunkard with his morning draught, they steady their shaking limbs by the use of morphia. And when the effect of the latter passes off, and the mental and bodily depression that follows makes them feel their sad and helpless condition (similar to. the misery that follows the abuse of spirits), and their morally and physically miserable life, they again and again make use of another injec- tion of this poison, in the hope of forgetting the misery partly brought on by themselves.

But the lucid intervals which allow them to lead an existence worthy of human beings become shorter and shorter; the craving for morphia increases daily; the vicious circle draws closer and closer around them, until, at last, all power of resistance having failed, they succumb under its action.

With regard to the state of the mind, the morbid craving for morphia has much resemblance to dipso- mania, even to the delirium, which will be hereafter described. Both diseases have the same pernicious form of inflammatory action on the lungs, the intes- tinal tracts, etc. They differ, however, in some important respects, inasmuch as our disease, contrary to dipsomania, selects its victims from among the higher and more educated classes of society, as there are no symptoms of fatty and amyloid degeneration of the internal organs, and as there is no mental disease showing itself during the poisonous action, with the exception of a rapid change of temper.

Another resemblance of our disease to dipso

mania is shown by our patients, male and female, not unfrequently becoming drunkards. Some of them use alcohol as a stimulant as soon as the action of the drug begins to abate; others pretend that their desire for alcoholic beverages is due to the experience that they then feel less wish to resort to morphia; while others, again, imbibe alcohol so as to endeavour to abstain from morphia altogether; but, nevertheless, they always fail. Even those who have recovered from the morbid craving for morphia retain a liking, and even an increased longing, for alcohol. They often, indeed, indulge in excessive drinking, and, finding that the newly acquired passion is more injurious to them in their social relations than the craving for morphia, they try to amend by recurring to injections of this drug, thus again succumbing to their old enemy.

According to Lähr[1] and Fiedler,[2] who were the first to draw the attention of the medical profession to the abuse of morphia injections, and who, in relating a number of characteristic cases, have proved the serious nature of this abuse, the morbid craving for morphia is a mental alienation.

I do not hold this opinion.

Every person, whether of a strong or of a weak constitution, has a tendency towards a morbid craving

---

[1] Lähr, 'Ueber Missbrauch mit Morphium-Injectionen,' *Allgemeine Zeitschrift für Psychiatrie*, 1872. Heft 3.

[2] Fiedler, 'Ueber den Missbrauch der Morphium-Injectionen,' *Zeitschrift für Medicin*, 1874, Nos. 27 and 28, and *Jahresbericht der Gesellschaft für Natur- und Heilkunde*, Dresden, 1876, p. 185.

for morphia, if from any disease he has become accustomed to injections of morphia, providing these injections were under his control

Consequently, the morbid craving for morphia injections ranks amongst the category of other human passions, such as smoking, gambling, greediness for profit, sexual excesses, etc. The desire for morphia injections, felt by all debilitated and nervous persons, who lack the power of resistance against it as soon as they have come to appreciate its effects, results from their natural constitution, and not from a certain predisposition for its use.

With respect to the state of excitement caused by the administration of morphia, we might easily be induced to classify the morbid craving for morphia among the mental diseases following intoxication, such as chronic intoxication with alcohol,[1] lead,[2] arsenic, and oxide of carbon. The latter, however, are caused by changes of the central nervous organs, while morphia only causes functional derangements; furthermore, mental disorders due to intoxication with alcohol, lead, arsenic, and oxide of carbon, last for months and years at a time; those produced by morphia disappearing again in a few hours.

Again, they differ from true mental disorders, inasmuch as the latter, as well as the derangements of the mind caused by intoxication, cannot be checked

[1] Böhm, 'Intoxication durch Alcohol' (Ziemssen, *Pathologie und Therapie*, tom. xv. p. 112).

[2] Naunyn, 'Vergiftungen durch schwere Metalle und ihre Salze,' *ibid.*, p. 278.

or modified in their regular course of development, even should all obnoxious influences and all the other causes of the mental alienation be entirely removed.

A mother who sinks into profound melancholy at the news that her sons have perished in the war, and has to be removed to an asylum in consequence, is not restored to her senses by being told that the report turned out to be false.

A merchant who has become insane through a sudden fall in the value of his shares and stocks, does not recover in less time if we show him the share list, and try to persuade him that the prices have risen again.

To describe the morbid craving for morphia as a mental disease it would be necessary, first of all, to show that the persons suffering therefrom are really impaired in their intellect and feelings. But this is by no means the case. I know a number of sick persons who suffer from morbid craving for morphia in a high degree, and who, at the same time, are not only in the full possession of their intellectual faculties, but who have risen to, and still hold, their place in the foremost ranks of science and art. Authorities in military matters, artists, physicians, surgeons, bearing names of the highest reputation, are subject to this craving, without the least detriment to their capacities.

Amongst other distinguished men, I particularly remember one who, up to the last moments of his life, was held in the highest admiration by the whole of the scientific world. Apparently all these men, in order to fulfil their professional and other duties, needed and still need the use of morphia as an agent to act upon their nerves, in order to maintain the necessary equilibrium of their intellectual faculties.

Surely we cannot deem a person insane whose mind or intellect never, or at least only for a few minutes or some hours, suffers from a slight aberration, but who is, on the contrary, mostly absorbed by his art or profession ; who fulfils his duties to his government, his family, and his fellow-citizens, in an irreproachable manner ; and who takes a warm interest in all that gladdens the human heart

The ill effects that show themselves after using morphia for a certain time, such as sleeplessness and other symptoms of reaction on the part of the nervous system, from its having been in an excited state for years past, only point to an over-exertion of a neurotic nature. Even the state of excitement attendant upon *chronic* delirium tremens, and arising principally after a temporary abstinence from the customary use of morphia, must only be looked at as disturbed nervous activity, not as a derangement of the mental faculties. They find their analogy in the state of mental anxiety, caused by diseases of the heart or blood-vessels, and by some affections of the respiratory organs.

With the fact once established that craving for morphia is not a mental disorder, any argument as to what form of alienation it belongs to is entirely out of question, and, least of all it can be compared (as it has been) to cerebral paralysis, because our disease is free from the principal symptom of the latter, *i.e.* dementia. The inability to keep away from the use of morphia, the apathy and giddiness while under the influence of it, are not to be taken as such. We should otherwise, by following this mode of judging mental conditions, soon be compelled to pronounce as insane every person subject to some hobby, or partaking from time to time of a narcotic or stimulant, and who, as the result of doing so, found himself either in an exhilarated or desponding condition.

The morbid craving for morphia, as a mental disease, can therefore have no legal importance; but we must except from this one symptom of the disease caused by the withdrawal of morphia: acute delirium tremens, which, like acute alcoholism, must be considered a mental disorder, as persons suffering from it are in a morbid state of derangement of their mental faculties, by which the exercise of their free will is entirely suspended.

SYMPTOMATOLOGY OF MORBID CRAVING FOR MORPHIA.

The symptoms showing themselves in morbid craving for morphia may be classified under these heads :—

 I. Symptoms of Chronic Morphia Poisoning.
 II. ,, ,, Abstinence from Morphia.

I. Symptoms of Chronic Morphia Poisoning.

The results arising from the abuse of morphia injections generally commence to show themselves after a period of from four to six months. There are cases, however, in which its deleterious signs only become evident after some years. The earlier or later appearance of the disorders depends upon the individual susceptibility, and not upon the larger or smaller doses of morphia administered in each case.

Many people afflicted with morbid craving for morphia feel quite well for a certain time whilst using the narcotic; no disturbances are felt, the appetite, and even the bodily weight, remains unaltered, while others become emaciated. Soon, however, a series of morbid appearances show themselves, originating in the cerebrospinal and sympathic nervous system. The different organs are affected in various ways : some are not implicated at all; in others, one distinct symptom predominates over others to such an extent as to be the chief cause of the patient's complaints.

The skin often loses its turgor, its previous colour, and its natural elasticity. The subcutaneous areolar tissue melts away, although some patients, especially ladies, retain a large quantity of fat in it. The face mostly becomes pale and ash-coloured, occasionally of a dark red hue; sometimes, however, it retains its normal colour; the perspiration frequently increases

to an alarming extent. Skin diseases are rarely met
with. Inflammation of the sebaceous glands, such
as zoster and similar eruptions,[1] which principally
affect the chin, the cheeks, and the intercostal spaces,
show themselves from time to time, disappearing and
returning again, in some cases to become permanent.
Abscesses and infiltrations of the skin show themselves at the places where the injections have been
made, extending sometimes over a large space. The
patients complain of cold, and even shiverings sometimes come on.

The eyes are often devoid of lustre, the patient's
glance is weak, miserable, and shy; after administering a new injection, however, they become ani-
mated, passionate, or enthusiastic. Double vision
and a diminished power of accommodation are not
rarely met with.

The pupils are generally contracted, frequently
disproportionate, rarely enlarged.

The mouth is generally parched, the patients
complain of being thirsty, there is nausea, vomiting,
dislike to meat, and want of appetite. The tongue
sometimes trembles upon being shown. The

---

[1] For reference about Herpes zoster, pemphigus, and other eruptions consequent upon poisoning (for instance, with oxide of carbon),
see Leudet, 'Arch. générales de Médecine,' 1865, vol. i. p. 513;
Charcot, 'Klinische Vorträge;' and Mougeot, 'Recherches sur quel-
ques troubles de nutrition consécutives aux affections des nerfs,' Paris,
1867. See also A. Eulenburg, 'Ueber cutane Angioneurosen,' Ber-
liner Klinische Wochenschrift, 1867, p. 203; and G. Lewin, 'Ueber
den Einfluss der Nerven auf die Erzeugung von Hautkrankheiten,'
Zeitschr. f. pr. Medicin, 1877, No. 2.

bowels are mostly confined; very rarely diarrhœa sets in.

The pulse in severer cases is very small, sometimes hard, but may also be thread-like. The only other symptoms observable on the part of the circulation and respiration are dyspnœa and palpitations of the heart.

The kidneys in severe cases secrete albumen. There is dysuria, and the quantity of urine frequently diminishes. The specific gravity of the urine is rarely very high. I have seen urines of 1·004–1·038 specific gravity, and the curious fact was that the urine of a patient possessing a high specific gravity at the first examination, showed the same until the end of the treatment, and *vice versâ*. It is but natural that there should have been some fluctuations, according to the quantity of urine secreted daily; but they still showed the above conditions when compared with the average quantity.

The urine of people afflicted with morbid craving for morphia will nearly always reduce an alkaline solution of sulfate of copper, not precipitating it as an oxydulate. At the same time, this urine generally turns polarised light to the *left*.

On the part of the organs of generation there is weakness, impotence, and only very rarely increased excitability.

The menstrual discharge stops through the habitual use of morphia.

The central nervous system will become affected

in many of its functions ; quarrelsomeness, want of
sleep, hallucinations, changeable temper, hyperæs
thesia, neuralgic complaints, paræsthesia, trembling
of the hands, and increased reflex action, are the
chief symptoms shown by these organs.

II. Symptoms of Abstinence from Morphia.

Although persons who suffer from morbid craving
for morphia show different symptoms, some of them
beginning to feel the effects of the poison after using
it for several months, while others enjoy comparatively good health for years together, there is no
difference between them as regards the consequences
upon the partial or entire withdrawal of the narcotic
drug.

In this respect they are all equal. None of
them have the power of satisfying their passions un-
punished.

Only a few hours have passed since using the
last injection of morphia, and already the feeling of
comfort brought on by the action of the drug is
passing off. They are overcome by a feeling of
uneasiness and restlessness ; the feeling of self-con-
sciousness and self-possession is gone, and is replaced
by extreme despondency ; a slight cough gradually
brings on dyspnœa, which is increased by want of
sleep and by hallucinations.

The vasomotoric system shows its weakness by
abundant perspiration, by the dark colour of the face,

which replaces the pale condition apparent during the first few days.

Flow of blood to the head and palpitation of the heart, with a hard pulse, soon show themselves. The latter symptom often disappears suddenly, and is replaced by a slow, irregular, thread-like pulse, which is a sign of the beginning of a severe collapse.

The reflex irritability increases, the patients begin to sneeze and to have paroxysms of yawning; they start if anyone approaches them; touching their skin causes crampy movements or convulsions; the trembling of the hands, if not already evident, now becomes distinctly perceptible. The power of speech is disordered; lisping and stammering takes place. Diplopia, and disorders of the power of accommodation, frequently accompanied by increased secretion of the lachrymal glands, show themselves. The patients are overcome by a feeling of weakness and total want of energy, and are thus compelled to lay in bed.

Neuralgic affections of various parts of the body, pain in the front and back of the head, cardialgia, abnormal sensations in the legs, associated with salivation, coryza, nausea, vomiting, and diarrhœa, tend to bring them into a desperate condition.

Some persons will bear up with fortitude under all these trials; they will quietly remain in bed, and will endure the unavoidable suffering, hardly uttering a complaint. Of the others, although the great

minority of them sleep and dose during this trying
time, some can find rest nowhere; they jump out of
bed, run about the room in a state of fear, crying
and shrieking. Gradually they become calmer, although occasionally their excitement increases. A
state of frenzy, brought on by hallucinations and illusions of all the sensitive organs, at last causes a
morbid condition, to which I have given the name of
Delirium Tremens, resulting from morbid craving
for morphia, it being similar to that caused by
alcohol. Some of the patients, however, will be
found walking about in deep despair, hoping to find
an opportunity of freeing themselves for ever from
their wretched condition.

CASES.

I. Normal Course of the Period of Abstinence.

Senior Lieutenant v. O., patient of Dr. T. Mayer, from Berlin,
32 years of age, belonging to a healthy family. First took to
morphia injections in 1871, on account of a gunshot wound received during the war. The largest quantity he used during a day
was 16 grains. Six weeks ago he began to abstain from its use,
but without any good result. Since the patient has used the
morphia he has suffered from want of appetite, constipation, and
impotence.

January 13, 1875.—**Sudden deprivation of morphia.**—
Patient has had no sleep; stumbles about the room. During the
day the restlessness gradually increases; patient feels uncomfortable in every position; moans and groans without ceasing; complains of cold, trembling all over, and nausea. There is much
yawning and sneezing. 3.30 P.M. had a warm bath of 28° R.
(82·4° F.), with a cold douche, and remained in it for a quarter of
an hour. After the bath the patient remained quietly in bed.

January 14.—Very restless during the night ; tremor of arms and legs. Patient gets up and stumbles as if intoxicated, moans, and asks for some alcoholic drink. This state lasted up to 4 A.M. Afterwards he becomes quieter. In the morning at 7.30 a bath with cold douche of half an hour's duration was ordered. After the bath he slept for a quarter of an hour. At midday he became very restless. 12.30 P.M. again a warm bath for a quarter of an hour with cold douche. In the afternoon he had several short naps. In the course of the day he vomited three times and was relaxed seven times.

January 15.—Patient has slept for two hours, vomited twice, been relaxed once ; otherwise the night has been pretty good. In the morning a warm bath (half an hour), which induced sleep. During the day relaxed twice; no vomiting. In the evening another bath with cold douche, which after half an hour gave sleep ; in the night, however, he was restless and fretful.

On the following day there was cardialgia and feeling of the iron band. Frequent sneezing and yawning, little appetite, four diarrhœic motions. Evening, 8.30 : quarter of an hour's bath with douche ; afterwards three hours' sleep.

January 18.—Patient has slept for three hours ; there is frequent sneezing.

January 19.—No sleep during the whole of the night, but much less restlessness. In the morning very little prostration. A bath with cold douche induced one hour's sleep. Pulse 72, powerful. Appetite good. In the afternoon relaxed once. He feels well in himself.

January 20. Only one hour's sleep. Patient awakes with great dyspnœa, paroxysms of yawning, feeling of anxiety, starting.

January 21.—Two hours' sleep. Bath with douche. 45 grains of chloral at night.

January 22.—Patient slept the whole of the night ; feels a little weak during the day ; is somewhat restless.

January 26.—Slept for three hours without chloral. Erections and seminal emissions have occurred.

Patient left the Institution on February 9, 1875.

The urine on being boiled with alkaline solution of sulphate of copper, except turning yellow, showed no abnormal condition. The average daily quantity of urine amounted to 1,000 cubic centimetres (about 1¾ pints), with a specific gravity of 1·012.

II. Normal course of the period of abstinence.
(Diplopia).

Mr. L. S., merchant, 30 years of age, was in 1869 treated with morphia injections, on account of neuralgia of both supraorbital nerves, which acted with such good effect, that the pains were soon removed. In the spring of 1871 there was a recurrence of the neuralgic complaint. From this time the patient administered the injections himself. A trial to do without them was unsuccessful, and Mr. S. at the time of his admission into the Institution used about 3 grains of morphia per day. In consequence of this his appetite became bad, the bowels were constipated, sometimes for five or six days, there was inaction of the detrusor vesicæ, the patient suffered from profuse perspiration, and his sexual power was diminished.

Present state.—Patient is short and stout, muscles and panniculus adiposus well developed. On examination of the lungs, heart, liver, and spleen, no complaint of any kind could be found. Weight, 122 pounds.

April 3, 1872.—**Sudden deprivation of morphia.**—Patient has had scarcely any sleep during the night. Some light pain is felt in the arms and legs, pressure and burning of the eyes, yawning. In the afternoon headache and great restlessness ; patient moves about in the bed, moans, and declares that he would never have undergone the treatment had he known that the pains would come on. Altogether he vomited twelve times and was relaxed fourteen times. Pulse regular.

April 4.—No sleep during the night ; pains in the calves of the legs and in the stomach, frequent shivering, yawning and sneezing. Face pale, skin dry. Vomited twelve times, relaxed eleven times. Palpitations of the heart and a reddened face show themselves. Patient has slept half an hour during the day.

April 5.—Shivering and heat occur alternately ; there is great thirst, pains in the legs. During the last 24 hours he vomited eleven times and was relaxed eleven times. Patient partakes of coffee, beef-tea, and wine. At night 45 grains of chloral were given.

April 6.—Patient has slept for five hours, feels weak ; he is still restless and fretful, shivering and sensation of heat still come on alternately, and there is still stomachache, yawning, sneezing, &c. Very little appetite. Altogether vomiting occurred twice and relaxation six times. At night 45 grains of chloral.

April 7.—Five hours' sleep; complains of stomachache, pressure on the eyes; has no desire for morphia. Shivering, yawning, and sneezing as before. During the night vomiting occurred once, during the day three relaxed motions. Appetite moderate. At night 45 grains of chloral.

April 8.—Has slept for seven hours, and feels pretty well in the morning; has vomited once during the night, and has passed three thin, pulpy motions during the day. Patient could already move about in fresh air for several hours in the course of the day.

April 9.—Patient feels well in himself. There is still a slight amount of trembling and pressure on the stomach. Diplopia has set in.

April 11.—The nights were good after taking a dose of chloral. Yawning, sneezing, and trembling as before during the daytime. Diplopia less marked and of little inconvenience. 30 grains of chloral given.

April 12.—One seminal emission during the night. Diplopia has disappeared, otherwise state the same.

April 14.—For the last two nights patient has not taken any chloral, and has in consequence had hardly any sleep. There is again a craving for morphia.

April 16.—Has had two hours' sleep in the night, one seminal emission; feels pretty well considering.

April 25.—Patient has felt well for the last few days, has slept well, has no craving for morphia. Weight, 131 pounds. He leaves the Institution May 1st.

There had been no relapse twelve months after leaving.

III. Normal course of the period of abstinence. (Slight collapse).

Mrs. A. W., patient of Dr. Seemann from Berlin, 40 years old, mother of two children, in the year 1865 suffered from concussion of the brain, which confined her to her bed for two months. Subcutaneous injections of morphia were resorted to on account of severe pain in the back of her head, and were administered by the medical attendant up to the year 1869. Two injections only were made daily. From this time the patient herself began to inject the morphia, so much so that in the year 1873 as much as 16 grains of morphia was used daily. She then began gradually to diminish the quantity used, until one grain of the morphia sufficed for the daily use, but was again soon compelled to take more, and at the time she came under my treatment (April 1st, 1876), was injecting six grains *pro die*. During the use of morphia the following symptoms became apparent : want of appetite, stomachache, constipation of the bowels, which were moved only every five or six days. Trembling of the limbs, chiefly during the night.

Great restlessness, delirium, and anxious dreams.

Present state.—Patient is short and stout built, with well-developed muscles and panniculus adiposus. Auscultation and percussion of the lungs, heart, liver, and spleen show no abnormities.

April 3.—Sudden deprivation of morphia.—Pulse irregular during the day, want of appetite, frequent yawning ; complains of head- and stomac-hache, pyrosis and nausea, itching in the limbs. Patient moans and is unhappy ; wants to interrupt the treatment, and to ride home.

April 4.—Patient has not slept during the night ; has been moving about in the bed moaning and shivering. Face presents a dark red colour. Frequent yawning and sneezing ; skin dry. Pulse from 60 to 80, and regular. During the day patient had hallucinations of smell ; in the afternoon languid pains in the legs and organs of generation ; very restless, vomiting. 40 grains of chloral which was given at night was again brought up.

April 5.—No sleep during the night. Vomited fourteen times during last 24 hours. Face of a red colour. Temperature normal. Continual shivering. Pulse varying and irregular. Thirst, and pains in the head and stomach ; great objection to light or noise. Patient has taken a little black coffee, some marsala, and champagne. She again brought up 30 grains of chloral given at night.

April 6.—Has had no rest during the night. Vomited eight times, relaxed five times during the day ; pains in the back and the limbs ; patient is somewhat less fretful. Pulse regular ; complexion brighter. The chloral given at night (40 grains) is again brought up.

April 7.—At three o'clock in the morning, after the patient had been very restless, a slight collapse took place. Pulse small and irregular, 132 beats. 72 respirations per minute. Face dark red. On being questioned, patient answered with difficulty, and in a slow manner. Has feeling of oppression and anxiety. The pulse and respiration become less turbulent, so that at 4.30 A.M. they are 100 beats and 24 respirations per minute. Nothing but champagne was given. In the course of the morning and forenoon the patient soon rallied, had some appetite, and felt pretty well. During the day she passed two thin motions, vomiting once. The food taken was coffee, milk, beef-tea, and wine.

April 8.—Patient has had hardly any sleep in the night, and much sneezing. At 9 o'clock in the evening 45 grains of chloral were given.

April 9.—Five hours' rest. During the day frequent shivering and pain in the hands and feet. Appetite good. Patient has been out of bed for a few hours. Five relaxed motions.

April 10.—Very little sleep. Pains in the head, back, and stomach. Vomited once. Appetite good. Relaxed three times. In the evening 45 grains of chloral.

April 11.—From six to seven hours' rest. Nevertheless feels very low ; complains of stomachache ; was relaxed six times. Appetite good. Got up for eight hours.

April 24.—Patient has slept on the average from three to five hours during the nights. Frequent sneezing ; health good.

On May 13 patient was discharged, sleep having become regular.

Some time ago patient paid me a visit. She now and then suffers from neuralgia in the face, but has had no return of the craving for morphia, notwithstanding this complaint.

IV. Normal course of the period of abstinence. (Increased reflex action—slight delirium.)

Mr. v. B., officer, sent to the Institution by Dr. Günther of Dresden and Prof. Westphal, suffered from an inflammation of the membranes of the spinal cord, caught during the war against Denmark, which became very painful during its progress. Frequent blood-letting, sulphurated baths, sea-bathing, galvanic treatment were all of no use, and he could only obtain relief from morphia injections. These not only allayed his physical pain, but also made him easy about his domestic affairs—the loss of his fortune and the separation from his home. Since then Mr. von B. has suffered from morbid craving for morphia.

The abuse of morphia soon induced sleeplessness, increased reflex action, hyperæsthesia, paræsthesia, neuralgic complaints, twitching of the muscles, dryness of the mouth. His face showed a deep red colour; he perspired on the slightest exertion, and often when resting quietly, to such an extent as to have to change his linen several times in the day.

This intelligent and highly educated gentleman had no inclination for any occupation whatever; he felt weak, prostrate, and altogether unwell.

Present state: Patient is of robust constitution; chest normal; face of dark red colour; pupils remarkably large.

July 18.—**Sudden deprivation of morphia.**—Face of dark red colour; mydriasis. In the forenoon patient had a bath of 20° R. (68° F.), and of ten minutes' duration. During the afternoon he felt uncomfortable, and started when his body was touched; complains of cold; there is much coughing, oppression, and sneezing. Relaxed motion. At 9 P.M. 45 grains of chloral were given. Very restless during the night; much coughing.

July 19.—Patient feels very weak this morning, and does not take notice of anything that is done near him; talks in a delirious, unintelligible manner; must be assisted about, and dressed after bathing. Relaxed motion; vomited. No appetite; had half-an-hour's sleep. During the afternoon he was relaxed twice; great prostration, vomiting. At 9 P.M. 60 grains of chloral were given. Half-an-hour afterwards patient had an involuntary motion in bed. There is slight delirium; he moves about in bed, and has very little sleep. Slight convulsive twitchings.

July 20.—Face dark red. Patient insists on having morphia. Stops in bed. Much sneezing; perspiration. During the afternoon several relaxed motions. At 9 P.M. 45 grains of chloral are given. Very little sleep during the night. Patient got up and dressed.

July 21,—Relaxed five times during the morning. Patient is too weak to be able to walk about alone. Pains in the lower part of the abdomen.

July 22,—Patient starts if only the door is opened. Dark red face; complains of abnormal sensations in several parts of the body. At 9 P.M. a bath of thirty minutes' duration, and at 28° R.

(82·4° F.), is given. Patient hardly slept at all, ran about the room.

July 23.—Vomiting, five relaxed motions, sneezing, yawning. At 9 P.M. a bath at 28° R. (82·4° F.), of thirty minutes' duration, and 45 grains of chloral were given. Patient slept till 11.30 P.M. and from 4 to 6 A.M. During the interval he ran about, knocked at the doors, and made a great noise.

July 24.—Patient felt languid in the morning, moans and groans, runs about, constantly hammers at the doors. Vomiting. After a bath he is somewhat quieter. Eight motions.

July 25.—No sleep, restless; ran about the room nearly the whole of the night. Seminal emissions. During the day he feels better, but is despondent and inclined to cry.

July 27.—Patient, after taking a dose of chloral, slept the whole of the night; in the day he felt weak and prostrate. Appetite good. His condition improved rapidly, and he left the Institution on the 16th of August in a cheerful and contented mind. He has since had a relapse.

V. Symptoms of abstinence with increased mental anxiety.—Unequal pupils.

Dr. R., medical practitioner, 30 years old, first injected morphia on account of neuralgia of the infraorbital nerve, but still continued the injections (3 grains *pro die*) after the pains were gone. Since that time patient noticed the following symptoms in himself: great feeling of weakness, profuse perspiration, five attacks of rigour, heat and sweating with no apparent type; a sudden heat and redness of the face, lasting several hours, came on occasionally; sexual instinct nearly gone.

Patient entered the Institution on the 26th April, 1876. Sudden deprivation of morphia. He is of middle size, well nourished, and of powerful and muscular build; pupils equal, not remarkably narrow.

April 27.—Patient has slept well. Pulse 64, strong and regular; **left pupil wider than the right.** During the afternoon shivering and heat alternately; restless manner, itching in the lower extremities, nausea, yawning, and sneezing. No appetite. Patient has not taken anything except a cup of coffee and a glass of champagne.

April 28.—Patient has had no sleep; vomited once during the night. Constant desire to move about. Pulse irregular; increased feeling of weakness and restlessness. Towards midday the face turned pale, twitching of the limbs, muscular quivering, mental anxiety; twenty minutes' sleep in the middle of the day. Patient cannot keep quiet in any position, whether in or out of bed. Relaxed twice during the afternoon, vomited once.

April 29.—Patient has had no sleep; relaxed twice, vomited once. Very restless during the day. Pulse 82, strong and full. Severe pains in the right calf up to the knee in the afternoon; relaxed twice, vomited once during the day. No appetite. 38 grains of chloral at night.

April 30.—Has slept from 9 till 12 o'clock at night; very restless after; severe pains in the back of the head; feels as if dying. From 2 o'clock headache, mental anxiety. Patient moves about in bed, taps on the blanket, talks incoherently, wants some morphia, wants to be carried to a lunatic asylum, as he is going mad. Pulse 48, strong and full. Face somewhat red, pupils middle sized, equal, react properly. At 9 A.M. headache and restlessness abate slightly. Stomachache, itching in the feet, frequent sneezing. Less desire for morphia. In the evening patient slept for three quarters of an hour; feels extremely weak; relaxed twice, vomited twice during the day.

May 1.—Vomited twice, relaxed once during the night. **Pupils unequal,** stomachache, depraved taste, much yawning and sneezing. During the day vomiting once, relaxation four times. In the afternoon patient was out in fresh air for half an hour; felt pretty well, had hardly any pain.

May 2.—Patient has slept for several hours; relaxed motion, frequent sneezing, one seminal emission; he felt pretty well, with the exception of having severe stomach.ache come on occasionally. Pupils equal.

May 3. — Hardly any sleep; relaxed twice, one seminal emission, frequent sneezing; rather restless in the night. Patient to-day feels weaker and more prostrate than yesterday; no appetite; shivering. A warm bath in the evening; pulse 72, strong. 45 grains of chloral at night.

May 4.—Seven hours' sleep. Erections in the morning. Patient feels well. Bath at night and 45 grains of chloral.

May 5.—No sleep; patient got restless and felt low spirited;

took again 16 grains of chloral at 9.30 P.M.; afterwards became excited, could not remain in bed, talked incoherently; said 'he felt as if the blood would burst out of his fingers.' Walked about the room till 1.30 A.M., muttering constantly; he then slept till 9 o'clock in the morning. On waking up he felt somewhat giddy; did not remember exactly what had happened in the night. He felt well during the day.

May 6.—Hardly any sleep (no chloral was given). Eyes heavy, speech imperfect, tongue trembles when shown. Feels well during the day, but in the evening is restless and prostrate. Appetite moderate.

May 7.—Two and a half hours' sleep. During the day very weak; appetite poor. 25 grains of chloral at night.

May 9.—Sleep regular; condition in the morning satisfactory. In the afternoon he became restless; feels weak and uncomfortable, has heat and shivering alternately. 5 o'clock a warm bath with cold douche. Pulse in the afternoon 128. 45 grains of chloral.

May 12.—Increasing restlessness towards the evening. Dyspnœa. Pulse 86. 45 grains of chloral.

May 13.—Restless and oppressed during the afternoon. In the evening urticaria shows itself on the hands and lower extremities. No chloral.

May 14.—Little sleep. In the evening dyspnœa, congestions to the head. Six leeches *ad anum* and a laxative were used. Urticaria gone.

May 16.—Sleep good without any chloral.

On May 24 patient was discharged in perfect health.

There was no albumen or sugar detected in the urine.

Patient has had a relapse.

VI. Gradual deprivation (Oliguria. Albumen during the period of abstinence)

J. S., in consequence of a coxitis of eight weeks' duration, had in his 13th year suffered from attacks of pain in the left leg, recurring at long intervals. For this in June, 1874, the first injection of morphia was administered; soon afterwards he made the injections himself, until at last he used the syringe thirty times a day (12 to 16 grains of morphia). Gradually want of sleep and appetite, pain in the abdomen, impaired urinary secretion, and complete loss of the sexual power came on.

Present state : Patient is of middle size, muscles moderately developed, pupils narrow, equal, react slowly after the direct influence of light. The physical examination showed wide-spread bronchial catarrh, and on this account gradual deprivation was resorted to.

August 26.—Two injections, each of 2½ grains of morphia, were given at night.

August 27.—Patient has slept pretty well during the night.

At 9 A.M. 2½ grains of morphia were injected.
„ 12 A.M. 1½ „   „   „
„   7 P.M. 1½ „   „   „

Complains of oppression of the chest and headache.

August 28.—Slept only till 12 P.M. Stomachache, trembling of hands and feet.

At 7 A.M. 1½ grains of morphia were injected.
„ 12 A.M. 1½ „   „   „
„   8 P.M. 1½ „   „   „

Appetite moderate, yawning and sneezing, rumbling in the abdomen.

August 29.—Patient has slept very little. Frequent yawning and sneezing, pressure in the epigastric region. Shivering.

At 7 A.M. 1 grain of morphia was injected.
„ 12 A.M. 1   „   „   „
„   7 P.M. 1   „   „   „

Pains in the back ; hands and feet restless, quivering of the sinews and muscles; great craving for morphia. Appetite moderate.

August 30.—No sleep after 11 o'clock last night. Frequent sneezing, pains in the abdomen, seminal emission.

At 6 A.M. ½ grain of morphia was injected.
„ 12 A.M. ½ „   „   „
„   7 P.M. ½ „   „   „

Feels uncomfortable, craves for morphia, weakness in the limbs. Patient moves about in bed. At 9 P.M. 45 grains of chloral.

August 31.—Patient has slept only from 11 to 2 o'clock. Very restless the other part of the night. Tearing pains in the limbs, principally in the feet.

At   7 A.M. 2½ grains of morphia were injected.
„ 12 A.M. 2½   „   „   „
„   7 P.M. 2½   „   „   ,,

In the course of the day he felt sick several times. Much moaning and groaning. Burning and itching in hands and feet. Mental anxiety renders patient's condition almost unbearable. In the evening at 9 o'clock 30 grains of chloral were given.

September 1.—Soon after taking the chloral patient became very excited and wanted to smash everything. Sleep very much interrupted. During the day he had eleven thin motions, and vomited seven times. Shivering, yawning, headache, and pains in the lumbar region. At 10 P.M. 45 grains of chloral were given.

September 2.—Hardly any sleep during the night. Vomited ten times, relaxed four times. Ran about the room moaning and groaning. Neuralgic pains in both extremities. Diarrhœa and vomiting also came on in the daytime. No appetite ; shivering now and then. At 9 P.M. 45 grains of chloral.

September 3.—No sleep in the night ; complains of severe headache ; muscular quivering, yawning and sneezing. Appetite poor.

September 6.—Patient has had no sleep during the past nights, although chloral has been taken. During daytime frequent sneezing, seminal emission, great prostration, lumbago. Appetite poor.

September 7.—Soon after having fallen asleep patient jumped out of bed and ran about the room in an excited state, dressed, complained of burning sensation in the hands and feet. During the daytime he felt comparatively well.

September 11.—During the past nights patient has had five hours' rest. Neuralgic complaints still prevail as well as sneezing and yawning. The appetite has somewhat improved. Bowels regular.

September 18.—Sleep regular. Pruritus cutaneus still persisting, gives him a good deal of trouble. General condition satisfactory.

September 27.—All the bodily functions are in a normal state. Patient left the Institution, and has had no relapse.

Urine.

August 26.—Spec. grav. 1·025. Reaction acid. Contains morphia, no sugar or albumen.

„   27.   „   „   1·028· Total quantity in 24 hours only 400 cubic centimetres, otherwise as before.

„   28.   „   „   1·029. Total quantity in 24 hours 560 cubic centimetres. Contains morphia.

·„   31.   „   „   1·010. Total quantity in 24 hours 975 cubic centimetres. Contains morphia.

September 1.   „   „   1·012. Total quantity in 24 hours 860 cubic centimetres. Contains morphia.

2.   No urine could be obtained on account of frequent diarrhœa.

„   3·   „   „   1·035. Quantity in 24 hours 435 cubic centimetres. Contains morphia.

„   4·   „   „   1·034. Quantity in 24 hours 530 cubic centimetres. Contains morphia.

„   5·   „   „   1·024. Quantity in 24 hours 705 cubic centimetres. Contains morphia.

Reaction Acid, Clear.

September 6.—Spec. grav. 1·021. Acid, thick. Quantity 825 cubic centimetres. Contains morphia.

„   7·   „   „   1·021. Acid, thick. Quantity 960 cubic centimetres. Traces of morphia.

„   8.   „   „   1·020. Acid, almost clear. Quantity 790 cubic centimetres. Traces of morphia.

„   9·   „   „   1·023. Acid. Quantity 625 cubic centimetres. No morphia.

September 10.—Spec. grav. 1·021. Acid, almost clear. Spermatozoæ. No morphia.

„ 11. „ „ 1·020. Acid, thick. Quantity 1,000
cubic centimetres. No mor-
phia.

„ 12. „ „ 1·026. Acid, clear. Contains epithelial
cells and a few spermatozoæ.
Small quantities of albumen.
Quantity 580 cubic centi-
metres.

„ 13. „ „ 1·020. Acid, yellow, a little cloudy.
Contained a small quantity
of albumen.

„ 14. „ „ 1·016. Cloudy, small quantity of
albumen.

„ 15. „ „ 1·019. Acid, clear, traces of albumen.

„ 16. „ „ 1·020. No albumen, no morphia.

VII. Gradual deprivation (amenorrhœa).

Mrs. von B., patient of Dr. Günther at Dresden and of Professor Westphal, 33 years old, was first treated with morphia
injection in the year 1865 for colic, caused by gall stones. She
continued the use for several months as soon as the attacks came
on. On the disappearance of the disease she left off the injections.

During the war of 1870–71 there was a fresh cause for using
morphia injections, as she resorted to them again, in order to try
to overcome the anxiety and worry about the daily dangers to
which her nearest relatives were exposed. During the last four
years she has daily used twelve grains of morphia. The symptoms
produced by the use of this drug were: hyperæsthesia, neuralgic
complaints and tertian ague. The menstrual discharge has stopped
for four years.

Present state.—Patient is a tall and strong lady, her face
is of a lead colour, the pupils are hardly as large as a pin's head.
All the organs accessible to examination are in a normal condition.

July 18, 1875.—The patient, who has accustomed herself to
use daily six to eight syringes of a solution of 5%, is only allowed

three syringes per day until July 21. The symptoms showing themselves during this time were increased reflex action, want of muscular power, feeling of illness, abnormal sensations in the skin, such as piercing and itching, and loss of sleep.

On the 21st patient was ordered 30 grains of chloral at night.

July 22.—At 2.45 A.M. patient had severe pains in the lower parts of the bowels, convulsive action of the limbs. Increased reflex action, pains in the urinary organs. Later on diarrhœa. She has not slept, and when in bed feels as if she is going to fall out of it.

Injection of $1\frac{1}{2}$ grains of hydrochlorate of morphia. In the afternoon twitchings in the limbs, very restless. Frequent sneezing ; complains of neuralgia in the bladder.

July 23.—Cries, and complains of pains in the region of the liver; feels very weak in the evening. Relaxed motion.

Injected $1\frac{1}{2}$ grains of morphia. At 9 P.M. 45 grains of chloral. Patient slept well.

July 24.—In the morning patient felt oppressed and giddy, had palpitations of the heart, and was very excited.

Injected $\frac{5}{8}$ths of a grain of morphia.

In the evening patient cried for morphia. The face is red, speech impaired. Relaxed five times.

July 25.—Patient was excited during the night, cried and groaned, ran about the room ; when she laid down, twitchings in the limbs at once set in. In the morning she vomited three times and was relaxed five times.

Injected $\frac{2}{3}$rds of a grain of morphia.

Patient cannot remember the events of last night. In the evening the same symptoms as yesterday are observable. After having taken 45 grains of chloral she slept pretty well.

July 26.—Until the evening the patient was moderately well. She only complained of having pains in the right hypochondriac region.

Injected $\frac{1}{3}$rd of a grain of morphia.

In the evening patient again became very excited. After taking 45 grains of chloral she slept till 4 A.M.

July 27.—Appetite good. Feeling of prostration, pains in the epigastrium. Relaxed motions. 45 grains of chloral.

Patient's condition is variable, especially as regards the temper. There are still occasional pains in the epigastrium and in the region of the liver, and diarrhœic evacuations. Patient feels uncomfortable; has a constant craving for morphia.

On August 11th the menstrual discharge reappeared suddenly, after having stopped for four years. From August 6th she slept without chloral.

On August 14, 1875, patient left the Institution in very good health. After a few weeks she had a relapse.

In comparing the symptoms brought on by the abuse of morphia with the pathological conditions for which the drug is therapeutically administered, the coincidence of both is very striking. Sleeplessness, hyperæsthesia, neuralgic complaints, mental anxiety, depression and excitement is combated as well as created by morphia.

In the same way the principal symptoms showing themselves in people suffering from morbid craving for morphia during the period of abstinence have the peculiarity of being soon removed by the use of morphia.

To show clearly the origin of the symptoms brought on by morphia and through being deprived of it, I have instituted a series of experiments on animals, which I shall enumerate at the end of each chapter of this work.

EXPERIMENTS ON ANIMALS.

I.

A small bitch was treated with subcutaneous injections of 1⅓ grains of morphia per day for nineteen days successively. Three to four hours after each injection we perceived *a rather profuse salivation, which disappeared again after a new injection.*

Urinary secretion very small, urine contained albumen. There was moderate desire for food.

On the twentieth day the animal died under general convulsions.

Post-mortem Examination.—Stomach full, mucous membrane of the stomach red and swollen. The intestines contained large lumps. In the kidneys, at the junction of the corticalis with the medullaris, there were, close to each other, two effusions of blood of the size of a lentil.

II.

A pigeon was treated with injections of morphia passed into the crop, $1\frac{1}{2}$ grains per day for six days, and was fed with fifty peas three times a day. For the sake of comparison another pigeon was fed in the same way, but morphia was not used to it. As soon as the crop of the latter pigeon was empty, both pigeons were fed with the same quantity of peas.

On the morning of the seventh day both pigeons had twenty peas, and four hours afterwards were killed by compression of the tracheal tube.

Post-mortem Examination of the Morphia-Pigeon.— The digestive tract taken out entirely shows the following condition: the mucous membrane of the œsophagus is swollen, the crop contains forty-two swollen peas. Its mucous membrane is covered by a quantity of grey, dirty secretion showing an acid reaction; the membrane in itself shows a dark red colour and a suffusion of blood under its entire surface. The muscular stomach contains the remainder of the peas. Contents and mucous membrane pretty dry.

Four minutes after the crop had been separated from its surroundings it showed a lively peristaltic action lasting for five minutes.

The post-mortem examination of the other pigeon showed an empty crop and stomach, no secretion in the stomach; the mucous membrane of the intestinal tract was in a normal condition.

III.

A pigeon was treated for twenty-two days with injections of morphia of a grain and a half per day. She finished the fifty peas given her in two days. On the twenty-third day she was found dead in her cage.

Post-mortem Examination.—The crop was filled with a detritus of swollen peas; the mucous membrane of the whole of the digestive tract was much congested and swollen. No secretion in the crop. Another healthy pigeon showed no abnormal condition after death.

IV.

A pigeon was treated with injections of morphia into the crop for thirteen days (a grain and a half daily), and thirty peas are daily forced into her stomach. On the afternoon of the thirteenth day the bird died.

At the post-mortem examination made immediately after death sixty-eight peas were found, having undergone no change. In the œsophagus there is a livid appearance all around its circumference; length, half a centimetre. The longitudinal marks at this part are tinged with blood. The dry mucous membrane of the stomach can be removed in its entirety. In the intestines there is a thin pulpy fluid. *The post-mortem examination of a healthy pigeon* shows a perfectly empty digestive tract and a normal mucous membrane.

V.

A pigeon with an empty crop is fed with seventy peas daily, and *an injection of a grain and a half of morphia per day is made into the muscles of the chest.* On the seventh day the bird was killed.

Post-mortem Examination.—There is a lively peristaltic action of four minutes' duration after the crop is separated. It contained fifty-five swollen peas. Its mucous membrane was slightly congested; muscular stomach filled with a great quantity of dry stuff; its mucous membrane dry.

The pigeon which served for comparison exhibited an empty crop and stomach and normal mucous membranes.

VI.

Five grains of morphia were daily given to a pigeon per os. Immediately after the administration of the drug the pigeon remains absolutely quiet, and allows itself to be touched without flying away. Eighty peas given at midday were eaten up; on the next day, however, peas could be distinguished by feeling the crop. Four weeks after, the pigeon was killed by compression of the tracheal tube.

Post-mortem Examination.—Crop perfectly empty, mucous membrane swollen, slightly congested, nearly dry ; the stomach contains numerous pieces of peas ; the intestines show fluid fæces.

The pigeon for comparison showed a perfectly empty intestinal tract.

VII

A large rabbit was subjected to daily injections of three grains of morphia for five weeks. There was very little craving for food, and the animal lost flesh. Urine was secreted every other day. *At the post-mortem examination* the stomach was found to contain food ; its lower part showed a livid mark of the size of a halfcrown.

VIII.

A pigeon was treated with daily injections of a grain and a half of morphia for five weeks, fifty peas being introduced daily, for the last time on March 15. The crop was always filled. On March 16 the bird died.

Post-mortem Examination.—Forty-nine peas, in different stages of digestion, were found. The muscular stomach contained a dry greenish detritus of peas. The crop after its separation showed a lively peristaltic action for two or three minutes. The mucous membrane of the crop and intestines were remarkably dry. The pigeon for comparison showed an empty crop and stomach, and normal mucous membranes.

IX.

A pigeon is treated with subcutaneous injections of three-quarters of a grain of morphia three times a day for ten days. Fourteen hours after the last injection, and after the last food of forty peas was given, the bird died.

Post-mortem Examination.—The crop, much distended with food, contained sixty-eight peas, partly swollen, partly crumbled up. The membrane of the crop was dry ; there was much detritus in the muscular stomach. Duodenum filled with pulpy fluid. Left ventricle of the heart much contracted ; the right

ventricle contained some coagulated blood. The pigeon for comparison had an empty crop and stomach, both ventricles of the
heart in diastolic expansion.

X.

A rabbit was treated with subcutaneous injections of
three grains of morphia daily for four weeks and a half.
The food given was cabbage and carrots. After a fortnight the
injections were stopped for two days. During this time lumpy,
pulpy masses were evacuated per anum; the urine contains albumen. Forty days after the injections were commenced, the animal
was found dead in its cage.

Post-mortem Examination.—The panniculus adiposus
had entirely disappeared. The heart had stopped during the
systole. Stomach entirely filled up, the intestines nowhere contain formed fæcal masses. The urine taken from the bladder
contains a pretty large quantity of albumen. The mucous membrane of the intestinal tract is very much congested.

XI.

A rabbit was treated with daily injections of two
grains and a half of morphia for thirteen days. The
animal passed very little water. Food was only taken in small
quantities, the bowels seldom acted, and the fæcal masses were
soft and pulpy. Died suddenly on the fourteenth day.

Post-mortem Examination.—Stomach filled with undi-
gested pieces of carrots; the intestines contain soft masses; their
mucous membrane very much congested, kidneys and liver the
same. The urine taken from the bladder contained albumen.

XII.

A middle-sized rabbit was treated with daily injections of three-quarters of a grain of morphia for four
weeks. The *emaciation* of the animal progressed from day to
day. The animal *lost its hair;* inclination for food diminished.

On the thirty-first day the animal was found dead in its
cage.

Post-mortem Examination.—Atrophy of the panniculus
adiposus. Stomach filled with half-digested food. The whole of

the intestinal tract contained thin fluid. The mucous membrane of the duodenum highly congested and slightly swollen, otherwise healthy. The urine taken from the bladder contains *albumen*, and after being removed it changes oxide of copper into oxydulate, turning the polarised light towards the left.

XIII.

A large rabbit was subjected to daily injections of one grain of morphia into the abdominal cavity. In the morning the animal eats part of its food, but does not take any during the course of the day. On the eleventh day after the commencement of the injection the animal died suddenly.

The post-mortem examination made immediately showed the following appearances: great emaciation ; the stomach is crammed with food ; the small intestines are in some parts contracted, the large intestines contain small quantities of thin fluid masses ; the mucous membrane of the whole tract is highly congested, showing on several places suffusion of blood. In the bladder there is bloody urine. The kidneys, microscopically examined, show no abnormal condition.

XIV.

A middle-sized rabbit was treated for a week with subcutaneous injections of two grains of morphia daily. Diminished inclination for food, and emaciation. *After eight days the administration of morphia is stopped. On the tenth day the desire for food returns,* and the animal eats double as much as before. The fæces, till then normal, become thin for three days after the use of the drug is done away with. The urinary secretion increases.

XV.

A small bitch was treated with subcutaneous injections of two grains and a half of morphia for twenty-seven days. The pupils, always of a *medium width before each injection, are contracted after the injection, and remain in this state. Reaction against the influence of light is diminished during this myosis.* On the second day after the drug had been stopped, *a remarkable difference in the size of the pupils was observed,* which however disappeared in an hour's time. A short time after each injection much salivation was noticeable.

The animal always took the food that was offered it. The usually very hard fæces now and then showed traces of blood. The urine from the third day the injections were commenced contained albumen.

XVI.

A small male dog was for the first ten days treated with injections of a grain and a half of morphia per day. The next day the quantity used was eight grains of morphia. Each injection brought on severe vomiting, as well as paralysis of the hind legs. During the time the drug was acting, there was myosis and evident paralysis of the recti interni. Very little desire for food. Urinary secretion retarded. On the fourteenth day convulsions of a tetanic character set in. Opisthotonus, spasmodic retarded respiration, pupils dilated ad maximum. Tracheotomy was at once performed and artificial respiration induced, so that the animal kept alive another fourteen hours.

Post-mortem Examination.—All the intestines were contracted, but still filled with food; the kidneys very much congested. The urine contained albumen, and showed a strong reduction of colour with Trommers's test, without, however, precipitating an oxydulate. The gall-bladder was in a turgescent state.

The deductions from the foregoing experiments are as follows :—

1. That internal application of morphia sooner paralyses the digestive powers of the stomach than the subcutaneous injection.

2. Both ways of administering morphia bring on functional disorders of the secreting nerves.

3. Both cause catarrh of the stomach and intestinal tract.

4. Large doses of morphia given internally cause a subacute catarrh of the stomach, on account of the irritating chemical action of the morphia.

5. The subcutaneous injection of morphia causes
a chronic catarrh of the stomach and intestines
in a mechanical manner, because in consequence of
the impaired influence of the secreting glands, due
to the action of the morphia, the secretion of the
digestive fluids is stopped altogether, or at least
diminished in quantity, and consequently the intestinal tract is encumbered for a longer time by the
ingesta.

The supposition that the action of the secreting
glands is diminished, or stopped altogether, by the
use of morphia is verified by an experiment of
Claude Bernard,[1] and by my own observations.

Claude Bernard, after giving morphia to a dog
and inserting a tube into the secreting duct of the
submaxillary gland, did not observe any secretion.
The shrinking and wasting of the mammary glands
of pregnant dogs and rabbits after continued injection
of morphia is a result of my own observation. —

This functional derangement of the digestive
glands also explains the respective symptoms of
morbid craving for morphia, as well as those noticed
during the first days of abstinence. The nausea,
vomiting, and constipation during the use of morphia
is caused by the chronic intestinal catarrh, which
although developing itself in a mechanical manner,
yet is later on a consequence of the paralysis of the
secreting glands.

---

[1] Claude Bernard: 'Leçons sur les Anesthésiques et sur l'Asphyxie.'
Paris, 1876, pp. 216, etc.

When during the treatment of morbid craving for morphia the drug causing the paralysis of the secreting glands is stopped, these latter are again stimulated to action. This sudden change, until the equilibrium is established, causes a superabundant secretion (increased flowing of tears, salivation, coryza). These as well as the alterations in the peristaltic action may be taken as the reasons, causing the stormy symptoms on the part of the digestive tract. The following experiment shows that an irritating or paralysing influence, on the part of those organs dependent on the sympathic nerves, must be explained by functional derangements of the central organs.

XVII.

For eight days three-quarters of a grain of morphia were given three times a day to a rabbit. Both ears and the conjunctivæ were of a remarkably pale colour. Conjunctivitis on both sides, as shown by a mucous and putrid secretion, abounding chiefly in the corners of the eyes.

After sharp friction of the ears the pale colour still remained. Temperature of the ears sensibly diminished.

The rabbit was tied down, a ligature was passed round the right sympathic nerve, and the animal was again released. Pale colour of ears and conjunctivæ unchanged. Closely watching the ears, the noose round the sympathic nerve was tightened. Almost at the same moment dilatation ad maximum of all the blood-vessels of the ear on that side was observable. The red colour continues, and the temperature is found to have increased when compared with the other ear.

The disorders of accommodation and of the muscles of the eye now and then showing themselves, in consequence of the abstinence, might be due to the respective muscles, which, paralysed previously by the morphia, are now regaining their former energy in a slow and irregular manner.

THE COLLAPSE.

On the second or third day after the deprivation of morphia a state of weakness in nearly all cases will supervene, due to the small quantity of food taken during the previous time, the diarrhœa, sleeplessness, and vomiting. The pulse gets small, the face becomes pale, the patient stops in bed and has the appearance of being utterly exhausted.

This slight collapse is of no great importance, and disappears as soon as the patient commences to take food regularly, or else it turns to a severe collapse, which is fraught with danger, and requires the greatest assiduity and care on the part of the medical attendant

The severe collapse may begin with premonitory symptoms, very often with a change in the voice and articulation. The patients are hoarse, they stammer or lisp when talking, there is twitching in some of the muscles of the face, and the trembling of the hands, already present, increases. The collapse may also appear suddenly at a time when the severest symptoms of abstinence, such as vomiting and diarrhœa, have passed off, and when we least expect such an occurrence. The patients while sitting in bed and talking to their attendants at once become quiet, fall back on the pillow, and sink into a state of unconsciousness, which cannot at first be overcome even by the most powerful stimulants. The face sinks in and is of a deathlike colour. The nose is pointed, the eyes sunk in, the bulbi rolled up, the respiration is troublesome, retarded, and gasping, the pulse can only be counted whilst listening to the heart.

In other cases the face is of a red colour, the eyes are bright, the pulse diminishes to 40 or 44 strokes, and the patient, after experiencing a feeling of nausea and approaching death, loses consciousness. If raised up the head falls on the chest, and no loud speaking or irritation of the skin is taken notice of. This condition may last from fifteen minutes to nearly an hour; it either recurs again three or four times during the twenty-four hours at short intervals, the patient in the meantime not entirely recovering his senses; or consciousness returns, at once; or, lastly, as observed by Fiedler [1] death ensues, accompanied by symptoms of paralysis of the brain.

CASES.

I. **Severe Collapse (Intermittent Fever, the result of Morbid Craving for Morphia). (Amenorrhœa. Changeable State of the Pupils.)**

Mrs. Jane G., a patient of Dr. B. Fränkel, of Berlin, 35 years old, eleven years ago, after having been suffering with typhoid fever, was afflicted with an abdominal complaint, which caused so much pain, that the family doctor had to administer an injection of morphia daily. Ten years ago patient married, and has given birth to two children, one five years, the other eight years old now. The confinements were protracted; both children died soon after their birth. During both pregnancies the use of morphia was

---

[1] Fiedler: 'Jahresbericht der Gesellschaft für Natur und Heilkunde.' 1876, p. 189.

discontinued by the doctor, the same taking place during several
occasional journeys to bathing places made by the patient because
of her complaint. For five years she has injected morphia herself, the largest dose *pro die* having been eight grams.

While using the drug a febris intermittens tertiana showed
itself two years ago, lasting, with an interruption of four weeks,
until November 1876. Regularly at 4.30 P.M. she had shiverings,
followed by burning heat, and ending in perspiration. The repeated use of quinine, even a change of air, and a sojourn in the
country were unable to suppress the fever. Dr. B. Fränkel, who
had only for three months attended Mrs. G., and whom she had
never told of her custom of using morphia regularly, made the
diagnosis of morbid craving for morphia only through considering
the intermittent fever. Apart from the latter, the use of the drug
had brought on the following symptoms: sleeplessness, headache,
principally in the region of the right occipital nerve, parched mouth,
loss of appetite, nausea, sickness, constipation, feeling of oppression,
mental anxiety, palpitations of the heart. Patient after having
hardly fallen asleep wakes up with dyspnœa, which increases to
actual fits of choking; swimming before the eyes and muscular
quivering.

Patient is admitted into the Maison de Santé, and the use of
the morphia is stopped forthwith.

October 16.—Hardly any sleep during the night; in the morning
patient is in a happy temper, makes no complaints. Temperature
and pulse normal. In the course of the forenoon there was much
perspiration, and patient complained of headache and nausea.
Pupils unequal, *the left smaller than the right.* Pressure on the
stomach, shivering, yawning; in the afternoon there is restlessness,
stomachache, epigastric pain, oppressiveness, much perspiration,
shivering. Poultices were applied to the abdomen. Up to the
evening she had altogether vomited twelve times and had one
relaxed motion. *Pupils unequal, the left wider than the right.*
The excitement in consequence of the pain in the stomach increases hourly. Patient moves about in bed and moans aloud.
Frequent spasmodic yawning. At 9 P.M. a bath with cold douche
of a quarter of an hour's duration is given, after which she became
quieter for a short time.

October 17.—Patient has been sick thirteen times during the
night; no sleep; the pains in the abdomen were very severe,

having the character of labour pains. Face pale, pulse 64, full, regular. Frequent yawning, burning in the throat, and abdominal pains continue during the whole of the day. Patient looks worn out, is now and then in a half-dozing condition. *Left pupil wider than the right.* Great prostration, great thirst. In the course of the day vomited nine times, two relaxed motions.

October 18.—No sleep during the night, restless; complains of tearing pains in the legs and excessive pain in the stomach; pulse and respiration normal; vomited four times, one relaxed motion, frequent sneezing during the day; she is very sensible to every kind of noise. Frequent retching; severe vomiting ten times. *Left pupil wider than the right.* Patient feels cold. In the afternoon at 5 o'clock patient lisps, becomes of a pale, deathlike colour, is very much oppressed, and loses consciousness; sinks back on to the pillows with closed eyes. Pulse 42, small, irregular. A quarter of a grain of morphia was at once given, and repeated after twenty minutes' time. *Right pupil wider than the left.* After a quarter of an hour patient wakes up, says that she had never felt so well before, takes milk with relish without bringing it up again. Pulse 60, strong and powerful. This favourable condition lasts till 9 P.M., when she again has nausea from time to time. At 10 o'clock a bath with cold douche is given.

October 19.—Patient has slept only from 10.30 P.M. to 1.30 A.M. At this time retching again occurs, vomiting, prostration, pains in the epigastric region; hallucinations, illusions set in, followed by collapse accompanied by the symptoms already mentioned, and necessitating the immediate injection of half a grain of morphia at 2.20 A.M., followed by a weaker injection of a quarter of a grain of morphia at 4.15 A.M. Afterwards patient again felt quite well. During the forenoon her condition has been good only at times, the principal complaints being great prostration, impossibility to sleep, pains in the stomach, great thirst. *Left pupil wider than right.* About 10 A.M. the sickness increased to such an extent that an injection of one-fifth of a grain of morphia had to be administered. Feeling well after it, patient partook of a pint of milk and soup. In the afternoon she had some cocoa, which she has not brought up. Towards the evening she felt oppressed, which however subsided after a warm bath with cold douche. At 9.25 P.M. another injection of a quarter of a grain of morphia had to be given on account of symptoms of a collapse showing themselves. Only three quarters of an hour afterwards the good effect was visible.

October 20.—Patient has slept altogether for five hours during the night, with many interruptions. During the intervals, besides being restless, there was prostration, craving for morphia, nausea, and frequent vomiting, and pains in the stomach. In the morning sneezing and yawning. During the daytime the condition was comparatively good. *Left pupil wider than the right, towards the evening the contrary taking place.* At 8.30 P.M. patient had a bath at 31° R. (87·8° F.) of half-an-hour's duration with cold douche.

October 21.—Restless during the whole of the night, craving for morphia and increased reflex action. During the daytime the condition of the patient is satisfactory, excepting some yawning, sneezing, and slight prostration.

October 22.—No sleep during the night, paroxysms of sneezing and yawning.

October 23.—Patient slept for three hours with interruptions. Towards the morning severe sneezing. Appetite good. She had a bath with cold douche morning and night.

October 24.—Patient was very restless in the night, moved about in the bed, and in the morning was much exasperated on account of the bad night. At 9 P.M. 40 grains of chloral were given in gruel, but were immediately brought up again.

October 26.—Patient slept for two hours with interruptions. During the remainder of the night she felt oppressed and had palpitations of the heart. Sneezing the same as yesterday.

October 28.—Very restless during the night. Patient had only about one hour's sleep towards the morning, and then felt pains in the lower part of the abdomen.

October 29.—Has had hardly any sleep during the night. Mental condition nevertheless good; appetite the same.

October 31.—During the past nights she slept on the average for three hours. Meals are taken regularly. 30 grains of chloral were given in capsules. Patient in the daytime complains of labour-like pains in the lower abdominal region.

November 1.—Patient slept for several hours after having taken 30 grains of chloral. The pains in the hypogastric region are still apparent now and then; some reddish watery spots show on the linen.

November 2.—The pains have increased in the morning; the whole abdominal region is sensitive to the touch. Poultices were applied. *In the middle of the day the menstrual discharge shows itself.*

November 3.—The pains have abated. Patient has slept for four hours.

November 4.—Menstrual discharge still continues. While it is said formerly to have lasted only for a few hours, it has now lasted for forty-eight hours. Towards midday the patient left her bed and remained on the couch for several hours.

November 5.—Slept from 11 P.M. till 2.30 A.M. Patient felt oppressed in the night, there was difficult breathing, and she could not remain in bed. Patient leaves the Institution on November 15, all bodily functions having become regular. She has up to the present time had no relapse.

II. Severe Collapse (Amenorrhœa, Albuminuria).

Mrs. von C., 33 years old, a widow, mother of two children, had been suffering from chloroosis since the age of puberty; the courses commenced in her 14th year. During childbed she had a putrid inflammation of the breast, followed by abscess, although she was not suckling the baby. To relieve the pains injections of morphia were administered daily. These were continued by the patient after the inflammation had gone. She injected daily 16 grains of morphia. In December, 1874, she was admitted into a hydropathic establishment for three weeks, in order to get rid of her practice of injecting morphia. Immediately after her admission the attendant physician reduced the injections to one administration at night, the strength of the dose not being known to the patient. At last he only injected water. As the patient could move about freely both inside and outside the Institution with her own attendants, she injected secretly during the night the same dose as before.

The principal complaints of the patient were : intense nervous excitement and sleeplessness, notwithstanding increased doses of morphia. Three years and a half ago patient lost her menstrual discharge and the fluor albus. Frequent headache, principally on the left side, diminished appetite, antipathy to meat, constipation.

For two years past she has suffered from attacks of fever, with shiverings and perspiration, having no regular type. She feels weak and lazy besides, has no energy, and is tired of life.

Present state.—Patient is tall and slender, pretty strongly built, has an abundant panniculus adiposus and pretty well developed muscles. Her attitude, manner of walking, and speech are normal. An eruption, resembling herpes zoster, has shown itself in the fossa mentalis near the place of exit of the nervus mentalis, as well as in the region of the nervus subcutaneus malæ.

The pupils react well under the influence of light, are middle sized, the left wider than the right. The chest and abdominal organs show a normal condition.

The urine contains albumen. The patient was completely deprived of the morphia. The course of the disease was as follows :—

November 11.—Patient has slept pretty well during the night. There were occasional abdominal pains. In the course of the day she complained of feeling sick and wanting to vomit, of shiverings and headache. Besides there is much yawning, perspiration, and increased lachrymal secretion. In the evening she gets restless, moves about in bed, insists on having morphia, and threatens to jump out of the window unless she is given some. Muscular quivering and pains in the abdomen and back. The skin is dry. The pupils do not react equally in the light, the right one gets contracted, the left one remaining the same. Temperature 37° C. (98·6° F.). At 10 P.M. 45 grains of chloral were given.

November 12.—Patient slept for two hours and three quarters; the rest of the time she moved about in bed in a restless manner. Insists on having morphia. In the day she feels cold, which cannot be removed even by wrapping her up in blankets. This is accompanied by nausea and four attacks of vomiting, and by pains in both calves; frequent yawning and sneezing, intense craving for morphia, great irritation in the throat, which makes her cough. In the afternoon she becomes quieter. At 3 P.M. patient suddenly turns pale, lies in bed with half-closed eyes, her head hanging down; she does not, if spoken to, answer questions; there is no sign to show that she hears anything that is said. Pulse 48, very small, respiration troublesome and deep. Pupils dilated ad maximum. Half a grain of morphia is injected twice, and after a quarter of an hour a third time. Marsala, black coffee with egg, and champagne, are administered at the same time, but with difficulty, as she strongly clenches her teeth. A mustard poultice is applied to the chest and water is sprinkled on her face. After several minutes she opened her eyes, but did not speak, and soon again sank into a state of unconsciousness, from which she could not be raised by talking to her. Face pale and sunken in. Respiration difficult and deep. This somnolence lasted until 4.45 P.M., then of a sudden she became lively, began to talk a great deal, and was very cheerful. This state lasted until 6 P.M. At five minutes past six she suddenly leant back on the pillows, closed the eyes, and did not answer when spoken to in a loud voice. Pulse remained strong. After cold applications to the head, marsala, and an injection of half a grain of morphia, she again recovered her senses. At 10 P.M. 45 grains of chloral in capsules were given, after which she slept off and on until 7 A.M.

November 13.—Patient felt well in the morning. About 9 o'clock she moaned and made some complaints, started suddenly after having closed the eyes for a few moments, asked where her father was, whom she had just seen and heard, raised herself up in bed and looked around in an excited manner; face red; the respiration all the while being difficult and spasmodic. After some time she earnestly begged to have some morphia or chloral, felt very weak, complained of shivering and abdominal pain, yawned and sneezed very frequently. Suddenly she became senseless, the pulse, in jerks, went down from 70 to 40. An injection of morphia of half a grain was administered. After that she felt well until 10 P.M.

November 14.—Patient slept with intermissions from 11 P.M. till 2 A.M. She then began to complain again of pain in the epigastrium, tearing pains in her legs, nervousness in arms and legs. In the morning she walked in the corridor for one hour, supported by a nurse. Towards the evening the craving for morphia became intense. At 9.30 P.M. 45 grains of chloral in capsules were given. The excitement produced by this drug, resembling for a time delirium, abated in the course of an hour. Patient slept very little, complained of pains in the legs and the epigastrium, yawned and sneezed a good deal. Temperature normal.

November 15.—There is a repetition of the abnormal sensations of yesterday; pressure and pain in the stomach, tearing pains in the legs, severe nausea, cold sensation in the limbs, and craving for morphia form the principal complaints.

A prolonged bath of 29° R. (84·2° F.) with cold douche is given.

At 10 P.M. patient took 30 grains of chloral in milk, and, after having at first become excited, slept only for short periods (half to one hour) from time to time. In the intervening time she would move about in bed, moaning and groaning.

November 16.—Shiverings, pressure and faint feeling in the epigastric region; painful sensations in the limbs predominate also this day until the evening. A bath of 30° R. (86° F.) from 7 to 7.30 P.M. She feels refreshed afterwards. At 9.45 P.M. she sleeps for a short time. Vomited. Slept several times for half to one hour with long intervals.

November 17.—Patient felt pretty well in the morning, later on the same complaints as yesterday. In the evening her temper was irritable. Among the symptoms of abstinence the sneezing greatly predominated. At 10 P.M. 45 grains of chloral were given.

November 18.—Patient has slept with intervals for six hours and a half during the night. Few complaints during the day. Bath from 5 to 5.30 P.M.

November 20.—After 30 grains of chloral patient has slept for about three hours; appetite has returned again. Increased secretion of tears. Bath from 10 to 10.30 P.M.

November 21.—After 30 grains of chloral patient slept for about three hours; felt well in herself.

November 28.—There is still little sleep. Paroxysms of yawning and sneezing sometimes occur.

November 29. Patient has only slept for about two hours, but feels well with the exception of a slight headache, which soon passed away. About 1 P.M. severe pains in the back and the left hypogastric region. She is relieved by a warm bath. Fluor albus shows itself.

Three weeks later the menstrual discharge appears, premonitory symptoms having shown themselves several days previously. The sleep improves, and the patient from this time enjoys perfect health.

Three months after her discharge I received information that the patient had not had a relapse.

The daily examination of the urine showed the following state: an average quantity of 950 centimetres, specific gravity 1·020, morphia could be detected until the seventh day after the abstinence. During the whole time the drug was stopped the urine contained a variable quantity of albumen.

III. Severe Collapse.

Mrs. H., 40 years old, sent to the Institution by Dr. Bernhard, has been accustomed to morphia injections for four years, using them at first on account of a neuralgic complaint. Daily use since last year, 12 grains. For the last year patient has complained of weakness, trembling of the hands, dislike to work, loss of sleep and appetite, constipation, mental anxiety, hyperhydrosis.

On November 18, 1876, at 7 A.M., the last injection of morphia was administered. At 12 A.M. restlessness, oppression, yawning; in the evening muscular quivering, extending over almost the whole of the body, and sometimes almost causing the patient to jump up; restlessness has increased, patient groans and cries, thinks she will die, sings sacred songs, preaches, and abuses the nurses. This state of excitement, intercepted by short periods of rest, continues till the morning with increasing intensity. Suddenly at 4 A.M. on the 19th the respiration becomes slower, irregular, and difficult; the pulse is weaker; the extremities are cold, her features look worn. This symptom of collapse is removed by two glasses of malaga wine and one glass of champagne. Soon afterwards vomiting comes on, followed by three hours of sleep. On waking up she is excited, there is muscular twitching, etc. At 8 A.M. while I was standing by the bedside, and after having answered my questions in a correct manner, although considerably excited, she suddenly became very quiet and talked unintelligibly; she does not now answer any more questions, there is no reaction when she is pushed about or called at, her eyes become fixed and are congested, the lower lip hangs down, the respiration is slow, and after a deep expiration her mouth fills with a foamy expectoration. The lips become livid, the face, previously red, is now pale; the pulse has sunk from 84 to 48, is irregular, soft, threadlike, trembling.

Treatment. After a morphia injection of half a grain, and repeated after a quarter of an hour, and douches with ice water are administered, patient recovers consciousness.

Towards the evening of November 19, the symptoms of abstinence show with increased severity. Vomiting, diarrhœa, stomachache, languid pains in the limbs, sneezing, restlessness, oppression, and craving for morphia continue during the whole of the night, the patient sleeping for about three hours with interruptions.

Otherwise the progress of the period of abstinence was similar to the cases related above. Patient soon regained her health.

DELIRIUM TREMENS, A SYMPTOM OF MORBID CRAVING FOR MORPHIA.

The delirium tremens brought on by morbid craving for morphia is accompanied by a series of symptoms bearing more or less the character of alcoholic delirium. Consequently the choice of this name does not require any justification; the same may be said of the morbid state called intermittent fever in consequence of morbid craving for morphia, as referred to hereafter, its symptoms being nearly the same as those connected with true malarial fever.

According to my observation, we may discern two forms of delirium tremens in morbid craving for morphia: the chronic, and the acute.

The delirium tremens chronicum is due to chronic poisoning with morphia, continuing into the period of abstinence, and not producing any mental excitement.

The delirium tremens acutum is only a symptom of the deprivation, and is accompanied by the most intense mental irritation.

The temper is of a changeable nature in the chronic form of delirium tremens. The patients are mostly of a jovial disposition, only occasionally interrupted by a short period of oppression. With some individuals the mental condition in the day-time is depressed; in the evening they become somewhat excited, and sometimes suffer from delu sions. Trembling of the hands and muscular quiver ing are a constant symptom of this kind of disease.

Notwithstanding this affliction, the patients are of sound mind, and perfectly conscious ; they may be roused for a short or a long time from their depressed or excited condition, and are able to take part in conversation.

The acute delirium tremens of morbid craving for morphia shows itself in the course of from six to twelve hours after the administration of the drug is stopped.

The patient at first gets fretful and restless, and constantly runs about the room, cries and screams, and at last, under the influence of painful sensations, becomes maniacal.

This state of mind, lasting only for some hours, is followed by a quieter condition, which is accom- panied only by hallucinations. These hallucinations are caused by all the sensual organs excepting the taste. They see birds of various colours, hear voices, feel as if sitting in the wet, and smell the most varied things.

Soon illusions of an hypochondriacal character supervene. The patient thinks he is dead, and has been present at his own funeral; the persons touching him, in his ideas, get taller and taller, etc., etc. Some of them will likewise talk to themselves, and carry on conversations with absent persons.

The trembling of the hands is increased, and is accompanied by muscular quivering, nystagmus, and tremor of the whole body.

At the commencement of the acute delirium, the voice and speech change in character.

This delirium tremens of morbid craving for morphia is not to be compared with a state of excitability also showing itself during the period of abstinence, which is caused by the administration of chloral.

If during the first two to four days a dose of 45 to 60 grains of chloral is given against the sleeplessness, some patients a few hours after its administration will become intensely excited. The patients cannot stop in bed, jump out of it, crying, laughing, singing, screaming, hammering at the doors and windows, knocking down the furniture, and at last begin to assault their attendants. Towards the morning they become quieter, and fall asleep for a short time, awaking generally with no recollection of the scenes of the night, so that the events which occurred can only be brought back to their memory with great difficulty.

The differential diagnosis of the delirium of morbid craving for morphia, from other delirious conditions, is only attended with difficulty if the original cause is kept back from the medical attendant, and if morbid craving for morphia comes under observation only in its latter stages, as then it is almost identical with chronic alcoholism in its principal symptoms, such as tremor, sleeplessness, slight impediment of speech, restlessness, mental anxiety, occasionally impaired sight, etc., etc.

The diagnosis also becomes more difficult if the patient suffering from morbid craving for morphia had lately taken large quantities of alcoholic drink, the latter fact only being mentioned to the medical attendant.

The difference between acute delirium tremens in consequence of morbid craving for morphia and the delirium tremens potatorum is as follows ·

1. The delirium tremens of drunkards is of spontaneous origin, or shows itself after traumatic accidents, or in the course of acute ailments ; the acute delirium caused by morphia becomes apparent only during the partial or complete deprivation of the drug.

2. In the acme of delirium potatorum the tremor mostly has gone, while it increases in the delirium of morbid craving for morphia.

3. Alcoholic beverages, often refused by the delirious person, increase the paroxysm, but never diminish or stop it; the patient delirious in consequence of the abuse of morphia asks for morphia, and becomes quieter for a short time after large doses of the drug have been administered.

4. The delirium potatorum lasts for several days or weeks. The duration of delirium tremens due to morbid craving for morphia lasts scarcely forty-eight hours.

5. The delirium potatorum ends in a collapse very often fatal, this collapse not being met with in delirium tremens of morphia poisoning.

A mistake with regard to delirium tremens resulting from lead poisoning[1] is hardly possible, as the gums show no greyish hue, and there is no paralysis of the extensor muscles in our disease; the change from excitable to a drowsy condition also excluding such poisoning.

CASES.

I. Delirium Tremens in consequence of Morbid Crav ing for Morphia. (Changeable Condition of the Pupils.)

Mr. F. H., 30 years old, private gentleman. On account of severe headache, lasting day and night for a long time, patient was recommended to use injections of morphia, which he administered himself. He began to inject in 1872, stopped the drug for a time of his own accord, but began again to use it towards the

---

[1] Wunderlich, 'Pathol. und Therapie,' tom. iv., p. 17. Griesinger, 'Pathol. und Therapie der psychischen Krankheiten,' 1871, p. 177.

end of the year, as the pains in the head were increasing, He gradually rose the daily dose of morphia to eight grains. When applying for admission to the Institution on October 29, 1875, he, according to his own statement, injected four grains daily. In consequence of the use of morphia he complains of the following symptoms : loss of sleep and appetite, constipation, diminished generative power verging on impotence, increased perspiration, attacks of fever (shivering, heat, sweating), showing no type, double vision, longing for alcoholic drinks, tremor of the hands.

Present state.—Patient is a tall, strongly built man, with powerful muscles and a moderate accumulation of fat. *Right pupil narrower than left;* auscultation and percussion do not show any abnormal condition of the lungs, heart, liver, and spleen. Urine contains neither albumen nor sugar, but much morphia, turns the polarised light to the left for more than two parts of the scale of the apparatus of Soleil-Ventzke.

October 30, 1875.—In the afternoon the treatment of deprivation was commenced. At 6 P.M. there was retching, restlessness, and craving for morphia. Patient took a great deal of wine. At 2 A.M. he jumps out of bed, says he cannot bear it any longer, if he was not better to-morrow he should kill himself; screams for morphia. *Breaks a door, again rushes back to bed,* moves about, swears and curses. The tremor has increased ; vomited once, one relaxed motion. At 5 A.M. *he talks quite incoherently.* He complains of severe epigastric pain, tearing pain in the limbs ; there is yawning, sneezing, shivering ; temperature normal ; pulse 72, strong and powerful.

October 31.—Patient does not exactly remember the events of the night, moans and groans, asks for morphia, gets restless, moves about in the bed. Shivering, yawning, sneezing, severe epigastric pains—' A perfect rumbling in the stomach.' *He again talks nonsense in the course of the day,* does not know that the doctor has visited him, sees double ; seven relaxed motions, and vomited twice. *Left pupil more dilated than the right.* In the evening tearing pains in the limbs, spasmodic contractions, very restless. At 9 P.M. 45 grains of chloral were given.

November 1.—Only one hour's rest in the night, very restless, craving for morphia, frequent yawning, sneezing, and thirst, complains of burning in the throat, violent pain in the limbs. In the morning one and a half hour's rest. At midday a warm bath with cold douche was given. At the least noise or touch, starts and feels a cold shiver pass all over him. In the afternoon a pain in the urinary passage when passing water. Towards the evening he becomes more restless. Severe pain in the epigastrium ; temperature 38·1° C. (100·58° F.). Great prostration ; he had five relaxed motions and has been twice sick in the last twenty-four hours. Pulse vacillates from 66 to 72, was hard and regular. At about 10 P.M. patient had 45 grains of chloral, which greatly excited him ; he jumped out of bed, ran about the room screaming and crying. At 11 P.M. another 30 grains of chloral were given ; he then rested from 12 to 1 A.M. Afterwards continual intense excitement.

November 2.—Patient screamed and cried in the night, was very delirious, fancied himself persecuted and betrayed ; towards the morning half an hour's rest. Seminal emission without erection took place. In daytime very restless, shivering, sneezing, yawning, head and stomachache, great objection to light, violent pains in the legs. Craving for morphia. Temperature 38·1° C. (100·58° F.). Eleven relaxed motions, vomited once. In the course of the day two warm baths with cold douche were given, the patient afterwards feeling a little better and quieter.

November 3.—During the whole of the day he was not very restless. There were periodical attacks of headache and pains in the stomach as well as cramp in the calves. Patient felt very weak, yawned and sneezed a good deal, but was able to spend an hour in the winter garden. Slept for several hours in the daytime with intervals. Pulse 60, full and strong, four relaxed motions, once vomiting.

November 4.—Slept for two and a half hours in the night with many breaks, suffered again from pains in the head, stomach, and calves, shivering and feeling of heat. Temperature normal. Pulse 64. Felt refreshed by the morning bath. Appetite moderate, eight relaxed motions, vomited once, frequent retching. The diplopia is now almost entirely gone, but he finds difficulty in reading, ' the letters get blurred.'

November 5.—Has slept for three hours altogether, again very restless, languid pains in the legs, severe headache, increased lacrymal secretion, and very sensitive to the light of the lamp. Much sneezing. In the evening patient feels comfortable.

November 6.—Hardly any sleep during the night, but not very restless during the first half of it. In the daytime the condition was tolerably good, excepting some pains in the epigastrium. Appetite good. Three relaxed motions. Frequent sneezing. In the evening 45 grains of chloral were given.

November 7.—Soon after the chloral was taken intense excitement came on. Patient throws himself on the ground, hammers at the door. Afterwards he slept for two and a half hours with intervals. During the day the condition is good. Appetite satisfactory.

November 12.—After having slept for nearly four hours in the night, he was in the morning in an excited state; speech hasty, quivering of the muscles of the face. Appetite good, bowels regular.

November 14.—Eight hours' sleep. In a very good frame of mind. Frequent sneezing, one relaxed motion.

November 24.—General condition satisfactory. Appetite, sleep, and digestion regular.

On December 6, 1875, patient leaves the Institution in perfect health. He has not had a relapse.

II. Delirium Tremens in consequence of Morbid Craving for Morphia (severe collapse).

Mr. von X., sent to the Institution by Professor Westphal, had caught cold while on a journey, which brought on rheumatic pains. To relieve him injections of morphia have been administered since 1872, at first by the medical attendant, and afterwards by the patient himself, and in increased quantities, the largest daily dose having amounted to 16 grains. The symptoms, showing themselves in consequence of this use, were loss of appetite and sleep, excited condition, emaciation, tremor of the hands.

On October 9, 1875, patient came into the Institution; he had injected morphia for the last time on the morning of the same day. At 10 P.M. patient went to bed and at once fell asleep. At 3.30 A.M. he was sick, felt very weak and prostrate, suffered from twitching in the lower extremities and diarrhœa.

October 10.—In the morning patient had five relaxed motions. Frequent vomiting during the whole of the day. Excitement,

and intense craving for morphia increases hourly. In the afternoon he talks of suicide.

October 11.—Patient has had no sleep during the night, but
has been frequently sick. Severe vomiting continued until 11 A.M.,
but stopped entirely during the rest of the day. Patient complains of languid pains in the legs, severe pain in the stomach.

October 12.—At 10 P.M. patient suddenly started up, and in
a frightened manner asked several times, ' Was not the doctor in
the room just now?' only the nurse having been present. Until
12 P.M. he laid in bed quietly without speaking ; he afterwards
raised himself up and screamed out in great excitement, ' Who is
that big fellow in the next room? He is so tall that he cannot get
through the door ! And now he is getting taller still. Now there
are several of them; they are ghosts !' His voice was trembling,
his extremities in constant convulsive movements. He was
quieted, but only with great difficulty. Again and again he raised
himself and anxiously looked at the door. Temperature 38·5° C.
(101·3° F.). In the morning the patient addressed the superin-
tendent as he entered as follows : ' Ah, good morning, dear Emily.
I am very glad you are coming !' Whilst saying so he was laying
down quietly. Now and then he raised his head slightly and
looked at the wall for a time, as if observing something, and his
lips were moving as if he was talking to somebody. In the course
of the day he vomited considerably several times. Patient feels
very weak, the speech is unintelligible, the tremor has increased.
He entered into a short conversation, and thinks himself better
than yesterday. Although very tired he cannot get to sleep.
Pulse was strong throughout the day. Auscultation and percussion
of the lungs and heart showed a normal condition. The bladder
was empty and no urine was passed until 5 P.M. Several relaxed
motions.

October 13.—Towards midnight patient suddenly raised himself
up, looked around, stretched his hands as if frightened, and called
out in a trembling voice, ' What do you want? There is the—the
ghost !' The voice next morning was hoarse, hesitating, unintelligible, devoid of sound. The features looked worn. During the
whole of the day there was diarrhœa and vomiting. An injection
of food into the bowels was given (after Leube).

October 14.—Patient has slept for only a quarter of an hour in
the night. The other part of the time he was dozing, vomited

four times, and had four relaxed motions. At 5 A.M. he called out to those watching him during the night, ' Come along, come along, quick, quick!' He gradually lost consciousness, did not move upon being called. Pulse 40, very small, hardly to be felt; respiration gasping, slow. Hippocratic face. Injected ¼ grain of morphia. Pulse and respiration soon became regular, and he regained his consciousness. There was no vomiting during the day. The voice is still gone, the features worn. Towards the evening the patient had an injection of food (Leube) of 16½ ounces. Great prostration. Skin moist and hot.

October 15.—Patient had no sleep, but lay quietly in bed until about 2 A.M., when there was vomiting, oppression, moaning, clonic contractions of the muscles of the face and extremities. Pulse strong.

October 16.—He had three relaxed motions, vomiting, and bleeding of the nose during the night. During daytime patient felt well.

October 17.—Patient has had no sleep during the night, but was quiet; vomiting and diarrhœa. In the day feeling of great weakness. Appetite good.

October 18.—No sleep, patient feels thoroughly knocked up. In the afternoon he slept for a short time.

From this time the patient's condition was satisfactory. He slept at first for three hours, afterwards for five hours, at last during the whole of the night ; the appetite increased considerably, the disposition was changed, so that he could leave the Institution on November 21st.

Urine.—The specific gravity of the urine vacillated between 1.019 and 1.029. A precipitation with alkaline solution of sulphate of copper was noticeable only occasionally.

The patient, whom I saw six months after his discharge, has had no relapse.

III. Delirium Tremens in consequence of Morbid Craving for Morphia (disordered speech, double vision).

Dr. X., physician, commenced practising injections of morphia on himself (daily dose from 8 to 16 grains), in order to overcome the worry and anxiety, which he caused himself through the undeserved self-accusation of having made a mistake in his profession. His senior physician told me that, in consequence of the use of the morphia, his previously very clever colleague had lost all elasticity, and that he was in consequence unable to give to the increased requirements of the service an increased bodily activity.   As the patient did not show any more interest in his duties, and as from his personal appearance he very often gave the impression of being tipsy, he was discharged from the medical service.   The morphia was withheld from him and narcein was tried as a substitute, but without avail.   On the morning of the fifth day of the abstinence he was found in bed holding a paper in his left hand, and with it going through unnecessary and automatic movements, either under the bedclothes or in the air.   He suffered from difficulty of speech, refused to take food, so that in his room one could already detect the peculiar sweet smell caused by one suffering from starvation.   He also had no sleep, was delirious, spoke of himself as of a third person, said that he had died and been present at his post-mortem examination, saw coloured and constantly changing birds, etc., etc.

To enable him to be removed to the Maison de Santé, larger doses of morphia were administered and renewed during the fifteen hours of his journey.   By these means he regained consciousness sufficiently to speak of his delirious state objectively ; but he was continually troubled by his hallucinations of sight and hearing. On his arrival here he stepped up to me in a friendly way, asked to be admitted, and answered my questions in a correct manner.

Present state.—Patient is of middle size and has moderately developed muscles, a normal attitude, staggers after closing the eyes, there is tremor of the hands, and he lisps when talking—as if tipsy, stammering now and then : " The pr-pr-pr- preacher there I think is-is doing business here in the pater-nosters."

One hour after the complete deprivation of morphia he began to be restless.   He insisted upon it, that he had been in a compartment with a princess, cried for morphia, screamed that his heart was perforated, hammered and kicked with both hands and feet against the doors and tables so much so that he had to be taken to the isolated part.   Here he screamed for two hours, said it was unjustifiable to treat him as a prisoner, abused the doctors and said they ought to know well how wrong such kind of treatment was, and that morphia ought to be used against his excitement.   By-and-by he became somewhat quieter and complained of shivering.   When asked to go to bed, he said that he could not undress as he was sitting in water, he even smelt the water ; then looked around frightened, and asked why the people in the corridor abused him in such a loud voice, and at last said he could see figures coming towards him in a threatening manner. The next morning at 6 A.M. patient was free from these hallucinations of hearing, smell and vision. He remembered them, and also the events of the previous day. The further progress of the illness was as follows :—

September 7, 1875.—Patient was again removed to his previous room, as he had become much more quiet.

September 8.—Patient has slept well during the night. He complains of shivering and of great discomfort, which however is not clearly defined ; yawning, severe nausea, relaxed motion. At 9 P.M. 45 grains of chloral are given.

September 9.—Has been quiet, but hardly slept at all. Frequent sneezing and yawning. Patient still lisps when talking.

September 10.—Patient was very restless, has slept little, power of speech better. At midday headache, nausea, sneezing and yawning. One relaxed motion.

September 11.—Slept for three hours and has otherwise been quiet, perspires, has pain in the front of the head, frequent sneezing and yawning, one relaxed motion, lisps. *Patient complains of seeing double and of being unable to fix an object.* Tremor and staggering after closing the eyes have disappeared.

September 12.—Patient has slept for four hours and a half with interruptions, feels well in himself, excepting great weakness. In the afternoon had a walk. Appetite good.

September 13.—Patient has slept for two hours only. Great weakness. Red face.

September 14.—Five hours' sleep with interruptions, much sneezing, prostration ; the face during the whole of the day still showed a red colour.

September 16.—Patient has slept for six hours ; he had erections and seminal emissions.

From this time up to his discharge the condition of the patient improved. Slept well without chloral ; all the other bodily functions returned and the interest for scientific occupation again showed itself to its full extent.

Urine.—The specific gravity of the urine varied from 1.036 to 1.022. The quantity averaged about 1000 cub. cent. Reaction was always acid. When treated with Trommer's solution the urine generally showed a reduction of colour without precipitating oxydulate of copper. One year and a half after the conclusion of the treatment patient had had no relapse.

INTERMITTENT FEVER IN CONSEQUENCE OF MORBID CRAVING FOR MORPHIA.

Intermittent fever, in consequence of a morbid craving for morphia, seems to be due to a certain neuropathic disposition, as it does not show itself with many patients, although they have taken large doses of the drug and for years together. It was, however, impossible to fix on any other cause for the development of intermittent fever but the use of morphia, as the respective patients lived in regions free from malaria, and as none of the other members of the family living under the same conditions showed any similar symptoms.

We may distinguish a light and a severe type of intermittent fever, when brought on by morbid craving for morphia. Both forms resemble real malaria fever, inasmuch as the first paroxysms, occurring at regular intervals, seemed to disappear after the use of quinine, returning, however, very soon, although the febrifuge was continually given; that, furthermore, they were improved by change of air, but came on again from the simplest causes, such as boating, errors of diet, etc.

The characteristic symptoms of this fever are the same as those caused by malaria : chilly feeling up to regular shivering, headache, oppression, heat and perspiration. They differ from one another in this respect that, immediately the morphia is discontinued, the attacks disappear without any treatment, although they may have existed a long time.

In some cases the intermittent fever sets in in an erratic manner. The patient at irregular times experiences an attack of fever with chill, heat, and sweating. These attacks recur from three to six times at long intervals, not showing themselves hereafter any more at all, or only after a great lapse of time.

In most cases the attacks of intermittent fever, in morbid craving for morphia, show a tertian, rarely a quotidian type. They are sometimes ante-, sometimes postponent. The attacks last from four to ten hours, and are followed by a normal condition.

The paroxysms disappear only in exceptional cases without the morphia being stopped. In this case the patients complain of experiencing an uncomfortable sensation, principally of an exhausting character, at the usual time of the attacks.

The feverish attacks are accompanied by neuralgic affections of the different nerves, principally in the region of the supraorbital, intercostal, and cardiac nerves.

The temperature is increased in all cases, varying from 38·5° C. to 40° C. (101·3° F. to 104° F.). The spleen is generally enlarged. The attack is followed by sediments in the urine.

In the severest forms of intermittens the patients get delirious when the fever has reached its maximum, cannot be kept in bed, and may become maniacal. Both forms cause great weakness and exhaustion, which last during the intervals.

CASES.

I. Intermittent Fever in consequence of Morbid Craving for Morphia.

M. H., law student, 24 years old, sent to the Institution by Dr. Ewald in 1874, was suffering from acute articular rheumatism when the first injection of morphia was administered. After his recovery, although not compelled to do so through pain, he continued the injections several times in the day, increasing the doses for the sole reason that he felt elated by them. The principal symptoms that resulted therefrom were, loss of appetite, progressive emaciation, loss of strength, and increased perspiration, which frequently caused the patient to become wet all over while in a cold room and quite quiet.

Before his admission into the Maison de Santé he was troubled with feverish attacks, which came on every two or four days, at different times in the day, in the following manner: first there was a chilly feeling for half an hour, followed by heat and profuse sweating. The latter was accompanied by the general symptoms of every feverish attack, enlargement of the spleen also being present.

Present state.—Patient is a tall, muscular man ; the examination of the internal organs shows no abnormal condition, excepting an enlarged spleen. Pupils of middle size, equal, reacting well. On December 10, 1875, in the afternoon, patient received the last injection of morphia.

December 12.—Patient slept in the night. In the course of the day he only feels a little sleepy. The face is red, the skin moist. Towards the evening there is nausea, pressure in the epigastrium, great restlessness, and stomachache. Patient moves about in bed, complains of headache, cannot get to sleep. Three relaxed motions.

December 22.—Patient has had no sleep during the night, three relaxed motions, vomited once. He complains of giddiness, restlessness and palpitation of the heart. In the morning there is a chill followed by heat and profuse sweating. Vomiting, diarrhœa. Until the afternoon he felt very prostrate and exhausted. Between 3 and 5 P.M. he got up. Soon, however, the symptoms of the morning return again, and pain in the knees, exhaustion, and restlessness compel him to go to bed.

December 23.—Has slept from 2 to 5 A.M. with interruptions. Profuse perspiration, nausea, intense craving for morphia, frequent paroxysms of sneezing. The sickness stopped in the course of the day. At 8 P.M. 30 grains of chloral were given.

December 24.—Only three hours' rest. Feels knocked up. One relaxed motion. Much sneezing ; craving for morphia. At 9 P.M. 45 grains of chloral were given, but were immediately brought up again.

December 25.—Patient has had hardly any rest. One relaxed motion. Has been sneezing frequently. Emission of semen. Great prostration, even in the horizontal posture ; red cheeks ; craving for morphia continues for the whole of the day. Appetite small. At 10 P.M. 45 grains of chloral.

December 26.—He has slept well during the night, only woke up two or three times. Pressure in the stomach, headache and palpitation of the heart come on now and then in the course of the day. At 11 P.M. 40 grams of chloral were given.

December 27.—Restless sleep, much interrupted. Patient went about the room, on waking up. During the day he complained of heavy pressure in the head.

December 28.—Patient has slept for about three hours. Sneezing. The red colour of the face of the past days was still present to-day. Although tired, he could get no rest. Two relaxed motions. In the morning a warm bath with cold douche was given.

December 29.—Patient has slept for nearly eight hours. Head not well yet. Severe sneezing. He feels better in himself. Towards the evening, however, an uneasy feeling came on in the legs. Three relaxed motions.

January 1, 1876.—Except the sleep being restless, patient feels well.

January 3.—Slept only from 3 A.M., ran about in a restless manner previously. Three relaxed motions. In the afternoon warm bath with cold douche.

January 13.—The bodily functions are all in a normal condition. General health good. There have been no further attacks of fever.

January 14.—Patient left the Institution.

He has had no relapse.

Urine. — The specific gravity varied from 1·012 to 1·020. Reduction of oxide of copper was noticed.

II. Intermittent Fever in consequence of morbid craving for Morphia. (Impotence. Disordered speech. Albuminuria.)

Captain B., sent to the Institution by Staff-Surgeon Dr. Peltzer, had been using injections of morphia in consequence of severe pains from a gunshot wound in 1871. For a time his medical attendant diminished the drug, but soon, by the advice of the latter, he purchased a syringe and bought the morphia, first at a chemist's, and afterwards at a shop where they sold chemicals ; he injected gradually as much as 24 grains per day. Several times his wife tried to stop the injections or at least to diminish the dose, but this was followed by vomiting, diarrhœa and loss of sleep, so that the doctor again recommended its further use.

The principal complaints of the patient on account of which he on December 20, 1875, sought admission into the 'Maison de Santé,' were ∶ the appetite is bad, the bowels are so much constipated that they are sometimes not relieved for eight days. From time to time patient suffers from disordered micturition, having to strain rather long before the water passes. Very frequently there was congestion to the head. and during sleep quivering of the muscles of the face and extremities. Now and then he suffered from giddiness and headache. He feels unwell, principally in the morning. Impotent for three years. He was obliged to resort to alcoholic beverages as stimulants, but he was no drunkard. From September 12 until the end of October, 1874, patient had had a shivering lasting two hours daily, followed by half an hour's heat and two or three hours' profuse perspiration. Large doses of quinine taken daily for a period of three weeks are said to have cured the fever ; it is worthy of notice that the patient stopped the use of the morphia during the latter period of the feverish attacks. Taking to it again, there was the same characteristic attack every week or fortnight at first; gradually, however, the free intervals became shorter, and at the time of his admission into the Institution the intermittens had again returned to the quotidian type. A treatment with large doses of quinine for several months, resorted to by his medical attendant, proved of no avail. Patient is pretty tall, muscles and subcutaneous areolar tissue very well developed. Face red. Eyes bright. Tremor of hands, slight degree of difficulty in speaking. Patient shows great vivacity in talking, his features move quickly, his movements are brisk. The physical examination of the thoracic and abdominal organs shows no abnormal condition, except a considerable enlargement of the spleen.

The morphia was at once withheld.

December 21.—Patient had a restless night, feels exhausted and knocked up; yawns, complains of cold, loss of appetite, severe headache on moving the head, and pains in the back; this is followed by nausea and at night by vomiting. Profuse perspiration.

December 22.—Patient was very restless in the night, got out of bed, ran about, laid down again, perspired freely, asked for morphia. The abundant perspiration lasted till midday and was accompanied by determination of blood to the head. Patient suffered from giddiness and felt greatly tired. Appetite poor. Frequent retching, but no vomiting.

December 23.—Patient has slept little. Three relaxed motions in the morning. Symptoms the same as on the previous day. New symptoms: twitchings in the extremities, excitement, sensitiveness to the light, and epigastric pains. To remove the latter symptom sinapisms to the stomach, hot poultices and cupping (four times) were attended with success. Frequent vomiting.

December 24.—Patient has only slept for a few hours. A great deal of sneezing, eight relaxed motions. In the course of the day he felt well.

December 25.—The pains and pressure in the region of the stomach have returned and he had also palpitation of the heart, was very much exhausted and suffered from tenesmus. Two seminal emissions.

December 26.—Four relaxed motions, shivering, feels uncomfortable.

December 28.—Patient has only had two hours' rest. Hands and feet burning hot. Eight motions ; during the day he felt weak, complains of formication in the hands and feet.

December 29.—Uncomfortable feeling continuing the whole of the day. Patient's face was of a dark red hue ; he complained of hyperæsthesia in the feet and of cold. Whilst reading a letter from his wife he began to cry, although the contents showed no reason for his doing so. Appetite good. Two relaxed motions.

December 30.—Slept from 3 to 7 A.M. Two relaxed motions. A great deal of sneezing, pressure in the epigastrium, appetite small.

January 3, 1876.—Slept from 12 to 4 A.M., after running about in a restless manner. Formication in hands and feet.

January 6.—General condition satisfactory. Appetite in creased.

January 14.—The patient has continued to recover his strength. Bodily functions normal. Sexual power has returned.

Urine.—During the first weeks of abstinence from morphia the urine contained albumen.

Patient left the Institution on January 22, in perfect health. He has not had a relapse.

THE AMENORRHŒA.

With all female patients whom I have attended for morbid craving for morphia, the menstrual discharge had become irregular, or had for months and even years entirely stopped. These ladies of from 25 to 35 years of age had injected large doses of morphia for a long time. The symptoms in the beginning and during the progress of the amen orrhœa, such as headache, giddiness, constipation, palpitation, hysterical fits, &c., are nearly the same as those produced by morbid craving for morphia, so that it sometimes is difficult to decide whether this or that symptom is caused by the poisonous influence of morphia or by amenorrhœa. I have never observed swelling of the breasts or bleeding from other organs during the cessation of the menses.

Amenorrhœa, in consequence of morbid craving for morphia, begins either with a dysmenorrhœa, or suddenly. Conception had never taken place in the above-mentioned cases ; a part of the patients had, however, become pregnant repeatedly before they resorted to the regular use of morphia. It seems probable, therefore, that the cessation of the menstrual discharge is caused by an anomalous condition of the ovaries, the latter becoming inactive.

According to Pflueger's theory, in cases of amenorrhœa due to morbid craving for morphia, the growth of the ovarian cells would be stopped from one monthly period to another, and consequently there would be a want of the stimulus on the ovarian nerves, causing on the one hand the rupture of Graaf's follicles, and producing on the other hand a congested state of the generative organs by reflex action. Hence the morphia would act in the same manner on the ovaries as on other secreting glands, i.e., would render them devoid of function under its continued influence. It is likely therefore that the menstrual discharge does not show on account of no ovulation taking place ; this also would account for the sterility.

The supposition that the functionary derange-

ment of the organs of generation is due to morphia
intoxication, is proved by the unmistakable fact
that the sexual power of female patients, suffering
from morbid craving for morphia, is again revived
after the use of the drug is done away with.

During the first period of using the drug, the
sexual instinct is increased, but is almost totally gone
(the same as with the male) when severe symptoms
of intoxication have set in. It is also worthy of
notice that ladies suffering from fluor albus often
lose their complaint after having taken morphia for
a lengthened period. It only returns again after the
withdrawal of the drug, and frequently shows itself
as an abundant discharge causing labourlike pains.

Ladies suffering from morbid craving for morphia, whose menstrual discharge is still of a normal
character, are able to conceive. But according to
my observations, the pregnancy only progressed in
the normal manner if the ladies used small doses of
morphia. They miscarried when using large quantities of the drug.

CASES.

I· Amenorrhœa. (Double vision. Different state of the pupils. Albuminuria during the period of abstinence.)

Mrs. von F., wife of a physician, 36 years of age, was hysterical when a girl, married when twenty years of age, and has given
birth to four living children and one stillborn. The fourth con-
finement, in 1872, was accompanied by an eclamptic fit. Since
then she has suffered frequently from mental anxiety, which was
combated by injections of morphia. Consequently since 1873 she
used to inject daily about 16 grains of morphia. During the use of

the drug the following disorders were noticeable : loss of sleep and appetite, constipation, amenorrhœa (since February 1874). Attacks of shivering, heat and sweating, occurring every eight days, lasting for 6 to 8 hours and disappearing without the use of quinine. Craving for alcoholic beverages (8 bottles of Bavarian beer per day). Patient is middle-sized, pretty dark and strong ; thoracic organs in a normal condition. Spleen enlarged. Patient who was admitted into the ' Maison de Santé ' on February 14th, 1875, states that she has not made an injection since last evening.

She is at once deprived of the drug. Until February 15th, 1875, in the afternoon, there were no symptoms of abstinence, a circumstance which did not coincide with the above-mentioned remark of the patient ; she eventually admitted having injected for the last time in the evening of the 14th, shortly before she rode to our Institution.

February 15, 6 P.M.—Pulse 84, moderately strong, easily suppressible, pupils equal, of middle size, react well. Towards the evening patient cried frequently, suffered from oppression and fear, had cold chills and feeling of heat. Increased restlessness, during the night, vomited once, very frequent sneezing. Patient is very unhappy, wants to go home. At 4 A.M. she is getting a little quieter.

February 16.—Pulse 54 in the morning, pretty strong, of moderate elasticity. *Right pupil somewhat more dilated than left.* Patient complains of oppression, respiration irregular. 7.30 A.M. bath of half an hour at 30° R. (86° F.). Until midnight, vomited 14 times, 8 relaxed motions. Restless, feels very much oppressed ; patient has no rest in any position, neither in bed nor out. In the afternoon at 5 o'clock pulse sinks to 48, is moderately strong ; the interval between each pulsation is not regular. Great prostration. About 6 P.M. patient became frightened, is restless, her face turning pale, pulse 48, small and of little elasticity, temperature 36·5° C. (97·7° F.). A cup of black coffee with some arrack was given ; hereafter patient became quieter and laid down. Pulse 48, a little stronger. In the evening patient still complained of restlessness; twitchings in the right arm and leg. Pulse 44 to 48, of moderate elasticity, pretty full. 8 P.M. warm bath of 30° R. (86° F.) for half an hour with cold douche ; while bathing one glass of marsala was given. After the bath patient was quiet for about half an hour. Frequent twitchings in the right arm.

February 17.—No sleep during the night, vomited four times, two relaxed motions. From 5 A.M. she became quiet; pulse 48, regular, respiration the same. Restless during the afternoon, twitchings in right arm and leg. Severe sneezing and yawning. In the course of the day she was sick nine times and had eight relaxed motions. *Double vision*, which prevents patient reading.

February 18.—During the night she slept from a quarter to half an hour several times, was sick once, not very restless. After a bath patient felt refreshed. Pulse 48, pretty full. *Right pupil larger than the left.* Complains of pains' in the stomach, restlessness, chills, weakness, languid pains in the legs. In the forenoon she slept twice for half an hour. During the course of the day vomited six times, four relaxed motions.

February 20.—About four hours' sleep with many interruptions ; diarrhœa, vomiting.

February 21.—During the night altogether two and a half hours' rest. Pulse 52, full, of moderate elasticity, no vomiting, no diarrhœa. *Double vision to a less extent.*

February 23.—**Diplopia still present**; when patient is reading, the letters get mixed up, and she is not able to fix them for any length of time. Had only one and a half hour's rest during the night. Appetite good, frequent sneezing. Pulse 60, full, of moderate elasticity.

February 26.—About 2 hours' sleep in the night. Feels well altogether. Appetite good. Bowels regular. About 7 P.M. an attack of palpitation of the heart and mental anxiety came on. Pulse 84, full, hard. After the evening bath with cold douche patient soon recovers.

February 27.—Little sleep. In the evening patients feels somewhat distressed. **No disorder of the vision.**

February 28.—Slept for several hours. There is still a good deal of sneezing. The patient cont'nues to feel well with hardly any exception. She left the Institution on March 18th, 1875, after having for several days past experienced some molimina menstrualia, the menses however not showing themselves. On March 18th, in the evening, at her own residence the menstrual discharge came on according to a communication from her husband.

Urine.—The quantity of urine during the period of abstinence was on the average 1000 cubic centimetres. On the fourth day it contained albumen, which, increasing for another four days, gradually diminished until February 22nd, after which date it was not traceable any more.

II. Amenorrhœa. (Collapse. Weakness of sight.)

Mrs. B. D., a physician's wife, 32 years of age, was when 24 years old and previous to her marriage, treated with injections of morphia on account of oppressiveness and mental anxiety.

At the time of her first pregnancy, 8 years ago, on account of sickness and faceache, injections of morphia were again resorted to ; she miscarried in the sixth month of her pregnancy. Since that time she has suffered from craving for morphia, using on the average 8 grains of morphia per day. Patient has had uninterrupted pregnancies 6, 4, and 2 years ago. The three children are living.

During the past summer patient suffered from a febris intermittens quotidiana. *For one and a half years the menstrual discharge has stopped.* The symptoms brought on by the use of the drug were as follows : loss of appetite, patient at last only living on milk and raw eggs. Constipation, sleeplessness during the night, drowsiness during the day. Profuse perspiration.

Present state : patient is slenderly built, possessing a moderate layer of fat. Pupils equal. Condition of the internal organs normal.

On September 18th at 7 P.M. patient received the last injection. During the night she had a few hours' sleep.

September 19, 1876.—Restless throughout the day, shivering, sickness. She gets up, but is soon compelled to lay down again.

Temperature normal. In the afternoon, severe yawning, paroxysms of sneezing, severe retching, fatigue, craving for morphia. A bath of 30° R. (86° F.) is given morning and night. The skin is moist. Pulse full, irregular. Respiration somewhat accelerated.

September 20.—Patient has had very little sleep during the night. Five relaxed motions. No action of the bowels during the day, vomited severely several times after taking milk. In the forenoon the patient's face suddenly turns pale, the pulse sinks from 68 to 48. She loses her voice, the tongue moves with difficulty, she is not able to keep her eyes open or to raise her head. There is difficulty of hearing. Pulse sinks to 44. *An injection of half a grain of morphia is administered.* Afterwards the pulse rises to

60 strokes per minute, still remaining irregular ; the eyes however become brighter, the hearing better, the weakness subsides. There was continued nausea and pressure in the region of the stomach during the day. Yawning and sneezing gone. She says that she is not able to see anything properly : all objects are getting mixed up. In the afternoon restlessness again came on, lasting until the evening.

September 21.—Patient has merely had one hour's rest during the night with interruptions ; she was very much excited, moaned and groaned, ran about the room, again laid down, soon jumping out of bed again. Pupils middle sized, *left more dilated than the right. Sight dim.* Eight relaxed motions during the day. Frequent vomiting. Yawning, sneezing, and retching. Great prostration. A warm bath with cold douche is given morning and night. Patient slept from 9.45 till 11.30 P.M. **Urine cloudy from a small quantity of albumen.**

September 22.—Patient was very restless during the night, so that she could only be kept quiet with the greatest difficulty. Two relaxed motions. Great wish for a bath, which she takes at 5.45 A.M. Chills and nausea. Bilious vomiting. Patient soon desists from a trial to read, as all the letters are said to get mixed up. Towards the evening she again becomes restless, has shiverings, nausea, and brings up bile in increased quantities. *Urine somewhat cloudy from albumen.*

September 23.—Restless during the night, slept only for one hour with interruptions. She takes beef-tea and milk, not bringing it up again. Six relaxed motions. Restlessness, shivering and severe sneezing still continues. Patient has been up for two hours.

September 24.—Patient has slept for two hours and a half, felt fatigued in the morning. During the day she feels better in herself. Patient walks about in the winter garden for a quarter of an hour. Disordered sight, sneezing and shivering still present. Two relaxed motions. The baths were continued.

September 25.—A good deal of sneezing. Patient cannot discern any objects properly.

Albumen in the urine not present any more.

September 26.—Patient slept for six hours with interruptions. The symptoms of abstinence are disappearing, excepting the difficulty of sight.

October 15.—Patient's condition until this day has been continually good. Since yesterday she has complained of pains in the stomach and back and of nausea.

October '17.—After taking her bath, the menstrual discharge came on this day. Pains in the stomach and back gone. The disturbance of sight has disappeared.

October 20.—Menstrual discharge has finished.

October 28.—Patient's health continues good. Bodily functions all in regular condition. She leaves the Institution on October 30th.

EXPERIMENTS ON ANIMALS.

I.

A pregnant rabbit with well-developed mammary glands is treated for ten days with injections of three quarters of a grain of morphia morning and night. On February 16 at 7 A.M. we found three dead rabbits and one still living, but breathing feebly. The latter died a few minutes after.

II.

A large pregnant rabbit is submitted to daily injections of three quarters of a grain of morphia for twelve days.

The animal took the food given to it several times in the day. On March 5 it gave birth to five dead rabbits.

III.

A large pregnant rabbit had 2 grains of morphia daily from March 18 till March 24. Took its food. On March 25 three dead rabbits were found in the cage.

IV.

A large pregnant dog was treated for eleven days with three daily injections of $\frac{1}{2}$ of a grain of morphia each. After four days a shrinking of the hitherto full and prominent mammary glands is observable. The animal took less food. Towards the evening paralysis of the hind legs regularly takes place (hyenoid walking, according to Claude Bernard). The mammary glands have shrunk still more, and after another week's time have dried up. The abdominal circumference has diminished. On the twelfth day the animal ran away, but came back after three days' time. She had most probably given birth somewhere to dead pups, as otherwise she would not have left them, or would have returned to them again.

V.

A small pregnant dog was submitted to daily injections of 2 grains of morphia for twenty days. At the time of the animal's advent the gravid uterus could be distinctly felt. The mammary glands were completely filled.

Under the use of the morphia the latter evidently became flabby and shrunken.

On the twenty-first day the animal at intervals of two hours gave birth to three dead pups, which, according to the opinion of Professor Hertwig, were in about the sixth week of their formation.

THE IMPOTENCE.

The experience of all the male patients, suffering from morbid craving for morphia, agrees in so far as they found an alteration in their sexual powers whilst using the drug. Either they have no sexual instinct, no voluptuous feeling, or the erections are incomplete, of too little energy and duration, or they do not come on at all. Thus these patients have suffered from sexual weakness in some cases increasing to complete impotence.

The larger proportion are those who give up sexual intercourse, or are obliged to do so for want of either personal inclination or of power, or through the want of complete or any erection at all.

Unmarried patients suffering from morbid craving for morphia generally become impotent sooner than married men, these latter having inducements tending to increase the sexual inclination that bachelors do not possess.

With many male patients the morphia will at first act on the genital organs in an exciting manner; later on, as already described, it paralyses them, and some unmarried patients suffering from this disease even take advantage of this latter experience, so that in case there should be any desire for sexual intercourse during a free interval, they overcome it by an injection of morphia.

The question in these cases also occurs as to whether there is any other cause, but the morphia, likely to have produced the impotence.

The state of despondency of many of our patients would perhaps justify the assumption of a psychical impotence; but on the other side we meet with patients suffering more or less from impotence, although feeling perfectly well, and the same takes place with others on whose psychical sphere the morphia has no influence whatever.

Whether it is the power causing erection that is first lost, or whether the function of the organs producing the semen is impaired previously (no seminal emission taking place in the severer cases), is not satisfactorily ascertained by the experience hitherto acquired. The statements of the patients suffering from morbid craving for morphia are not generally to be relied upon. Many will avoid talking of their impotence. If healthy persons are untrue in this respect, either exaggerating or concealing the fact, how much more so will this be found with people suffering from morbid craving for morphia, who are usually devoid of truth in all statements regarding themselves.

Looking at the register of admission of the ' Maison de Santé,' regarding the patients suffering from morbid craving for morphia, I find the remark entered that none of the wives of those gentlemen using large doses of the drug (16 grains) have gone through the full period of pregnancy during the last two years, although they were young and had annually given birth to children and never at an undue time before their husbands got accustomed to the drug.

I only relate these facts without drawing any conclusions from them, as the experience on this subject is at present based upon very slight material.

THE ALBUMINURIA.

I have frequently found albumen in the urine of patients suffering from morbid craving for morphia.

(1) During the continued use of the drug.

(2) During the period of abstinence.

The albumen showing itself during a continued use of the morphia injections is either a transitory symptom appearing in an irregular manner and observable often merely for several days, or it is of constant occurrence, only disappearing weeks or months after the complete withdrawal of the drug.

The albumen during the period of abstinence is observed much more frequently than the former, and occurs in nearly all cases ; it is first discerned from the 3rd to the 6th day after stopping the administration of morphia, disappearing again after some time (two to four days). It varies from slight cloudy deposits to flaky sediments.

Until cases of the latter variety came under my observation, I thought the slight cloudy appearance of the urine due to accidental admixtures, caused by slight catarrhal affections of the urinary system, but the sediments proved without doubt that pathological alterations were taking place in the uropoetic system.

In submitting these urines to chemical analysis[1] all re-agents, such as nitric acid, acetic acid, carbolic acid, ferro-cyanide of potassium, acetic acid, and sulphate of soda, promptly indicated albumen.

In some cases the reaction of the urine with nitric acid was remarkable, and reminded us of the case of Bence Jones[2] with its acid albuminate. The urine, to which a good quantity of nitric acid, was added,

---

[1] In analysing the carefully filtered urine of a rabbit, a slight cloudiness was seen after boiling and adding nitric acid. One of my younger friends, Dr. Ludwig Lewin, who happened to be at my laboratory at the time that I was occupied with this examination, and to whom I had spoken of the occurrence of albumen in the urine of people afflicted with morbid craving for morphia, said that he did not think this cloudy appearance was due to albumen. He filtered the fluid through charcoal, and there was no trace of albumen in the filtered residue. As, however, the existence of albumen in this urine to my mind admitted of no doubt, I considered that charcoal must possess the power of absorbing albumen. This supposition was proved correct by the following experiment :—diluted serum of blood and albuminous urine from a child afflicted with scarlet fever, after filtration through charcoal, showed no trace of albumen. *Charcoal therefore possesses the power of absorbing diluted albumen.*

[2] *Vide* Neubauer and Vogel, 1872, p. 89.

was heated ; there was no albuminous precipitate as long as the urine was warm, but it showed itself as the urine cooled, and disappeared again when heated afresh.

After it had been proved that the urine of patients suffering from morbid craving for morphia contained albumen, the question had to be decided whether the albumen was really caused by the use of morphia. The answer was in the affirmative, because the respective patients came into the Institution not suffering from any discernible disorder which could account for the formation of albumen, but only showing the usual symptoms of morphia intoxication, and later on of abstinence ; moreover, the connection between albumen and morphia was shown conclusively by the patients gradually losing the albumen after the administration of the drug was stopped. However, to remove any possible doubt, I made special experiments on animals, which I will relate after the enumeration of the following cases.

CASES.

I. Albuminuria during the use of morphia and during the period of abstinence.

Dr. Z., surgeon in the army, thirty years of age, used morphia injections, as late as March 1873, on account of sleeplessness brought on by the worry of the service, the dose at first being small, gradually, however, raising it to 10 grains per day. Since this time he observed in himself the following alterations :—sleeplessness, loss of appetite, craving for alcoholic beverages, constipation, emaciation, profuse perspiration, impotence, albuminuria.

During the year 1874 there was pretty frequently an atypical attack of chill, followed by heat and sweating. Patient entered the 'Maison de Santé' on August 27, 1876. Sudden deprivation.

Patient is tall, strong, and muscular, his thoracic and abdominal organs show no abnormities whatever. Pupils equal. Urine contains a large quantity of albumen.

August 28, 1876.—Slept well in the afternoon, some eructation, and retching. Perspiration. Shivering. *Left pupil more dilated than the right.* In the evening he twice vomited some slimy fluid.

August 29.—Patient gets gradually more restless during the night ; he at last leaves his bed, throws the pillows about, insists on having morphia, states his intention of discontinuing the treatment, and of starting on his journey to-morrow. Severe retching, vomited three times, one relaxed motion. Towards 8 A.M. the restlessness again increases. Pale and sunken face. Pulse 52, irregular, full, strong. Patient takes plenty of port wine, constantly wants to drink. Pupils equal. Sneezing, tingling in the ears, chill, itching in the limbs; very fidgetty. Patient is groaning continuously, asks either to have morphia given to him or to be discharged, etc., etc. There is a burning sensation when making water, abdominal pain, pressure in the region of the stomach. (Cataplasme instantané.) Until 9 P.M. twelve relaxed motions, severe retching, vomited twenty times. Pulse 44. Face sunken in, great bodily prostration. Treatment : two injections of morphia of ½ grain each. Pulse and strength are improving.

August 30.—Restless. Frequent yawning and sneezing. Twitching of arms and legs, quivering of the tendons. Towards the evening the restlessness increases, patient asks for morphia, has alternately a feeling of chill and of heat. *Pupils middle-sized, left more dilated than right.* 7.30 P.M. warm bath of a quarter of an hour's duration with cold douche.

August 31.—No sleep. Patient was restless, and suffered at times from severe stomachache. Three relaxed motions, vomited three times, paroxysms of sneezing. Two seminal emissions. In the morning craving for morphia. Pulse 60, full, regular. At 7.30 P.M. warm bath with cold douche. Ten relaxed motions, vomited once during the course of the day.

September 1.—Two relaxed motions during the night, about four hours' sleep with little interruption. Patient was not restless and had no pains. Three relaxed motions in the daytime. Much sneezing.

September 2.—Two and a half hours' sleep, two relaxed motions, restlessness. In the morning a warm bath with cold douche ; one and a half hours' sleep. Patient has a sensation as if an iron band was tied round the abdomen in the umbilical region, chiefly on the left side. When writing his hand trembles. Three relaxed motions in the day.

September 3.—Slept from 10 P.M. till 2.30 A.M., afterwards he was quiet until the morning. Sensation of the iron band much better. Sneezing. In the morning a warm bath with cold douche was given. Pulse 72, full.

September 4.—Two relaxed motions. Feels well but slightly fatigued in the legs. One pulpy motion. In the evening headache.

September 10.—Patient feels well, sleeps, has a good appetite, bowels regular, no restlessness. There is still a difference in the condition of the pupils, as well as sneezing and yawning. Frequent erections. Was discharged on September 26.

The *urine* on August 28 was of reddish yellow colour, slightly dull, a little acid, quantity 2420 cubic cent. Spec. gr., 1.006, contained a great quantity of albumen, no morphotic elements.

August 29.—Spec. gr., 1,007, quantity 2350 cubic cent. There still is albumen.

From August 30 the *urine* did not contain any albumen. —

II. Albuminuria during the use of Morphia.—Varying Condition of both Pupils.

Dr. G., medical practitioner, was in 1874 afflicted with suppurating inflammation of the skin, which, having been neglected, led to a phlegmone extending from the neck to the sternum. To alleviate the pain thus caused, morphia was first given internally, and afterwards by subcutaneous injections, from the autumn of 1874 till August 1875, at which time, so as to get rid of this custom, he submitted to a cold water treatment, but with no avail. From the time that he stopped the drug until November 1875 he became a drunkard. He drank twenty tumblersful of ale, sometimes more, daily. As he thought the injections of morphia to be the lesser of the two evils, he, in November 1875, again began to inject, and continued to do so until his admission into the Institution. The highest daily dose was 16 grains.

The symptoms arising from the use of morphia and alcohol were :—diminished sexual power, slight paralysis of the bladder. Hyperhydrosis. Appetite defective. Constipation. Supraorbital neuralgia. Loss of sleep. Since last year patient had atypical attacks of fever with chill, heat, and sweating. Albuminuria.

Patient is of middle size, pretty strong, with an abundant deposit of fat in the areolar tissue. Puffed and swollen face. Both pupils, equally wide, do not react very effectively. The examination of the heart and lungs shows no abnormal condition.

January 12, 1876.—At 12 A.M. patient had the last injection. In the afternoon there is already some restlessness and inability to lay down. Face red, pupils unequal, *the left more dilated than the right.* Increased sensibility. Two relaxed motions. At 11 P.M. patient went to bed but could not sleep, got up again and cried for morphia. Sneezing, five relaxed motions, vomited three times. Until five in the morning, pains in the legs, stomachache, headache.

January 13.—Patient feels prostrate, face pale, skin moist. Craving for morphia, sensations of chill and heat until 10, P.M. Vomited seven times, eight relaxed motions. Patient is for the greater part of the day lying in bed with closed eyes and does not like to answer questions. Pulse irregular. In the afternoon he complains of sickness, retching, pains in the abdomen and great restlessness. Strong quivering of the muscles. *Right pupil more dilated than the left.* Frequent sneezing and yawning, principally in the afternoon. The urine contains albumen.

January 14.—Patient slept from 11 P.M. to 1 A.M. From this time and during the course of the day he was eight times sick, and had seven relaxed motions. Patient lies quietly in bed, has little inclination to talk ; epigastric pains, frequent sneezing, great prostration.

January 15.—Patient has not slept in the night. Four relaxed motions during the night, the same in the daytime. Patient feels pretty well during the day, excepting great weakness and shivering in the limbs. Pupils unequal, *left more dilated than the right.*

January 16.—Patient slept from 12 to 1 A.M. He had thirteen relaxed motions up to the evening. Sneezing.

January 17.—Patient slept from 9.30 to 12 P.M. From this time until the next evening at 10 o'clock twenty-one diarrhœic motions and one attack of vomiting. Patient was very restless in the day, complains of feeling cold, of weakness, pressure and pain in the epigastric region, frequent sneezing, stomachache. (Cataplasms.) Pupils unequal, *left more dilated than the right.* The urine contains albumen in great quantity.

January 18.—Patient slept for five hours with interruptions. Both night and day there was increased appetite. He feels well in himself. Frequent sneezing.

January 19.—Patient slept from 10 to 12 P.M., and from 6 to 7.30 A.M. During the intervening time he was very restless, felt uncomfortable. Seven relaxed motions.

January 20.—Patient slept very little and was restless. Seven relaxed motions. Appetite good. Pupils equal. 45 grains of chloral.

January 21.—Patient had four hours' rest with interruptions. Appetite good, two pulpy motions. The urine contains small quantities of albumen.

January 22.—Patient sleeps well from this time without chloral. The albumen is gone.

Patient leaves the Institution on January 25. The quantity of urine passed during the period of abstinence was on the average moderate. Specific gravity, 1·025.

III. Albuminuria during the use of Morphia, and the Period of Abstinence. (Eruption in the Intercostal Region, similar to Herpes Zoster. Salivation. Double vision.)

Dr. X., medical director of a hospital, thirty-nine years of age, married, was at first induced to use injections of morphia in 1870 on account of a neuralgic complaint, and continued them with an interruption of eight weeks (during which time he took 5 drachms of Tinct. Opii Sx. pro die) until June 1876, injecting daily on the average 25 to 30 grains of morphia.

As early as half a year after commencing the use of the drug, symptoms of morphia intoxication, such as disordered digestion, fever, cramps in the muscles of the calves, and perspiration set in; since 1874 he has suffered also from impotence, paralysis of the musc. recti interni and of the bladder, the amelioration or aggravation of the latter being directly in relation to the quantity of morphia used ; at last he was afflicted with intermittent fever, first of a tertian, afterwards of a quotidian type.

Patient is tall, pale, and weak, has no energy, is tired of life ; his panniculus adiposus is well developed. Tremor artuum.

The skin shows an eruption, which has existed for one year, extending along the eighth intercostal space, and, excepting the want of pain, shows the characteristics of Herpes Zoster. Heart and lungs normal. Spleen enlarged. Urine contains albumen.

June 17.—At 10 P.M. patient has the last injection.

June 18.—Sleep good, 'although interrupted. Slight perspiration. **Strong Salivation.**—Weakness, trembling of the limbs.

June 19.—Patient has slept during the night, with frequent interruptions. Six relaxed motions in the day. Skin moist. Sneezing and vomiting. Double vision. The examination of the eyes *shows that he sees double at a short distance, not when fixing objects far distant. Fixing at a distance of twelve inches shows a slight divergence of an essentially dynamic character, but getting more perceptible after continuing the trial for a longer period of time. The insufficiency of the musc. recti interni is doubtless the cause of this divergence. The extent of the power of accommodation is smaller than one-twelfth, i.e. greatly diminished.*

June 20.—Slept little during the night. Patient was laying in bed quietly. Appetite moderate. Frequent paroxysms of sneezing during the day. Six relaxed motions.

June 22.—During the last two nights patient slept for five hours on the average. His general condition is somewhat better. The urine contains albumen.

July 13.—Patient sleeps on the average for about six hours. His appetite has increased. The bowels are still relaxed now and then. Sneezing and yawning have not yet left the patient.

July 20.—The intercostal eruption is healing gradually. Sleep and appetite normal. The other bodily functions are in perfect order.

July 21.—Patient leaves the Institution. He has had no relapse till now, and fills his position with the previous energy.

Urine.—From the day of patient's admission into the Institution the urine was examined daily. The quantity on the average was moderate, the specific gravity being at first 1·006, rising after three weeks to 1·014. For about three weeks there was a great quantity of albumen discernible, which diminished gradually, but did not entirely disappear until four months after the commencement of the abstinence. No morphotic elements could be traced. Alkaline solution of sulphate of copper was reduced by it, but not precipitated as an oxydulate of copper. Notwithstanding the loss of albumen, his weight during the five weeks of his stay had increased by eighteen pounds.

IV. Albuminuria during the use of Morphia.

Mr. P., Dr. Juris, gentleman farmer, sent into the 'Maison de Santé' by Professor Przibram, of Prague, thirty-seven years of age, married, father of three healthy children, has since 1873 been using injections of morphia against a neuralgic affection of the testicles. During the first four weeks he was sick every time he used the injection. Soon, however, patient got accustomed to the drug.

During the first year of the use of morphia, he felt very well, was almost always of a lively temper, and, according to his own saying, was more capable of work than before.

For the last two years patient himself noticed the following symptoms: he gradually lost his appetite, so much so that he could only take one third of the food that he previously took. Antipathy to meat. He was generally constipated, but as soon as he stopped the morphia, if only for a short time, his bowels became relaxed. The sexual power was greatly diminished. During the autumn of 1875 two attacks of shivering, followed by heat and perspiration, showed themselves in the course of three or four days, no repetition of them however taking place. Patient suffered repeatedly from palpitation of the heart, principally after injecting large doses. The urine contained albumen.

The highest dose patient pretends he has used was 8 grains per day. Patient has tried several times to stop the drug—at first in 1874, while staying at a cold water establishment. Showing however the symptoms of abstinence, the doctor there gave him morphia, which was followed by maniacal excitement for half a day. Patient pretends that he did not take alcoholic beverages at that time.

At the end of November, 1875, while on a railway journey, he attempted suicide with morphia. Soon, however, he felt remorse, telegraphed to the doctor of the next station for an emetic and brought up part of the drug. He arrived at his destination suffering severely. The truth of a second attempt at suicide may be doubted. Patient having been out hunting, came home with marks of small shot in his face, saying that some one else had wounded him through carelessness.

On December 21 patient for a second time submitted to a treatment of abstinence at his own residence. At 7 A.M. he had the last injection, eleven hours later he is said to have had shivering, increase of temperature, a tiny pulse, collapse, dyspnœa, mental aberration. He was relieved by an injection of morphia.

On December 25, renewed trial of abstinence. Shivering six hours after, symptoms not so severe, temp. 37.4° C. (99.32° F.), perspiration, spasmodic swallowing, which necessitated the administration of morphia. Patient now decided on entering the 'Maison de Santé.' During the journey there he had morphia every four or five hours, was very restless, took off his clothes ; there were periodical attacks of mental aberration. Last injection of morphia at 11.35 A.M. He was admitted into the 'Maison de Santé' on December 29 at midday.

Present State :—Patient is a tall man of considerable strength, with a good panniculus adiposus. Walks carelessly, bending forward. Colour of the face grey. Pupils middle sized, equal, react properly. Spleen not enlarged. The examination of heart and lungs shows no abnormal condition. There is a varicocele on the left side.

December 29.—Appetite good, in the evening patient partook of several glasses of wine. Face rather puffy ; yawning ; micturition attended with difficulty. At 9 P.M. patient takes 45 grains of chloral, sleeps very little, has no rest while in bed, his walk was unsteady and staggering. Pains all over the body. No albumen in the urine.

December 30.—Patient has been sick four times and had twenty-eight relaxed motions during the day. Pulse, respiration and temperature normal. After a warm bath with cold douche he slept for a few minutes, and again during the forenoon. He began again to be restless after, there was pressure in the epigastrium, nausea, chill, piercing pains in the region of the heart ;

tenesmus, groaning and crying for morphia. The epigastric pains increased, principally after the vomiting. At the same time profuse perspiration sets in. Patient is not able to walk about the room. No albumen in the urine.

December 31.—Nine relaxed motions. Vomited twice. Frequent sneezing. The symptoms of yesterday continue. Left pupil somewhat more dilated than the right. In the course of the day patient now and then slept for a quarter to half an hour.

January 1.—Patient had three warm baths with cold douche in the course of the day and at 10 P.M. 45 grains of chloral. During the first part of the night he was very much excited and restless. Later on he slept for four hours with interruptions. There is again restlessness, epigastric pain, yawning and retching. Twenty-two relaxed motions, vomited nine times. Appetite moderate.

January 3.—Patient slept in the night without any chloral. Sneezing, yawning, epigastric pain and restlessness are again apparent to-day. Twenty-eight relaxed motions and nine attacks of vomiting. Temperature and pulse normal. Three warm baths with cold douche.

January 4.—Neither diarrhœa nor vomiting; the restlessness and pressure in the epigastrium have diminished; patient complains of pain in the thigh; all the food he takes has to him a nasty taste and smell.

January 5.—Patient slept for four hours and a half with interruptions. In the morning severe paroxysms of sneezing, pain in the thigh and upper part of the arm. Appetite has returned. At 9 P.M. patient takes a bath for half an hour at 30° R. (86° F.). The restlessness and inability to remain in bed hitherto observable left for a short time. Soon, however, they returned again. He suffered from palpitations of the heart and headache, moans and groans, has nausea.

January 6.—Patient has had two hours' rest. During the night the first erection showed itself. Patient is unable to read for any length of time. Appetite good.

January 7.—Patient had not slept in the night. Until midday he felt pretty well; in the afternoon prostration again came on; palpitation of the heart, retching, sneezing. Appetite good.

January 8.—No sleep during the night. One seminal emission. General condition good during the day. At 9 P.M. 60 grains of chloral were given. Slept for six hours.

January 9.—After a warm bath with cold douche patient slept for one hour and a half. One seminal emission. A walk in the afternoon made the patient feel uncomfortable and nervous.

January 11.—During the morning pains in the thigh ; in the afternoon patient felt comparatively well.

January 20.—The neuralgia in the thigh, after having been treated with the constant current, disappeared. Sleep sufficient.

Patient is discharged on January 20. No relapse.

The average daily quantity of urine was 1,800 cubic centimetres, with a specific gravity of 1·018. Morphia could be traced in the urine until the sixth day after withdrawal of the drug.

V. Albuminuria (Varying Condition of the Pupils. Febris Intermittens).

Sister Mathilda, deaconess of a hospital in Westphalia, was in September 1870 afflicted with articular rheumatism, and has become accustomed to morphia since. She injected daily 16 grains, and raised the dose so as to use it as a stimulant in case she felt weak and fatigued by her trying profession. Until 1874 the morphia had caused no special inconvenience to her health ; soon, however, febris intermittens tertiana, accompanied by delirium during the time of the attack, came on. This fever, which the attending medical man could not account for, as malarial disease had not before been observed in that part of the country, and as the treatment with quinine was of no use, was *intermittens in consequence of morbid craving for morphia.* Patient had her last attack two days before her admission into the Institution.

Since 1874 she has further suffered from want of sleep, loss of appetite, pain in the epigastric region, constipation, emaciation, hyperdrosis, paralysis of the bladder, and palpitation of the heart. For one year the menstrual discharge has stopped.

Patient was admitted into the Institution on March 24, 1876. She is of middle size, pretty well nourished. Face red. No abnormal condition is noticed on examining the thoracic and abdominal organs. Spleen not enlarged. Pupils unequal, *the right more dilated than the left.*

As patient felt very much fatigued from her journey hither,

the proper treatment could only be resorted to on the third day after her arrival; until then the previous dose of morphia was injected.

On March 27, 1876, the morphia was suddenly withdrawn.

March 28.—No sleep, very restless during the night. Patient could not remain in bed; much nausea, frequent sneezing, face slightly red. Feeling of formication in all the limbs; restlessness, shivering, sneezing, abundant secretion from the mucous membrane of the nose. Six relaxed motions, vomited three times. *Pupils dilated, right more so than left.* In the afternoon *the right pupil is more contracted than the left.* Pulse 52, regular, strong; stomach-ache and pain in the epigastrium. Twelve relaxed motions, vomited four times. At 10 P.M. 30 grains of chloral were given.

March 29.—No sleep, vomited twice during the night. Seven relaxed motions accompanied by pains in the abdomen and arms. Sneezing. *Right pupil contracted in the morning, more dilated than the left in the afternoon.* Fifteen relaxed motions, vomited three times during the day. Pains in the lower part of the back, sneezing; face red.

March 30.—Very restless in the night, only half an hour's sleep. Seven relaxed motions, headache. sneezing, languid pains and twitchings in the calves; nausea. Disagreeable taste in the mouth. Burning in the soles of the feet. Less pain in the back and stomach. Singultus. *Right pupil more dilated in the morning, more contracted in the afternoon than the left.* Eleven relaxed motions, vomited once. 30 grains of chloral.

March 31.—Three and a half hours' rest, three relaxed motions during the night. Patient felt weak, but got up for a short time in the afternoon. Complains of burning in the hands and soles of the feet. Frequent nausea, paræsthesia of the taste. *Double vision* when reading. Pulse 64-72, irregular, pupils differ almost every hour; *in the morning they are equally wide, at 1 p.m. left more dilated than the right, at 3 p.m. right more so than the left, at 3.30 p.m. both equally wide, and at 7.30 p.m. right again more dilated than left.*

Vomited once, seven relaxed motions in the day, 30 grains of chloral at night.

April 1.—One and a half hours' sleep. Restless. Pruritus in the palms of the hands and the soles. Epigastric pain. Bad appetite. Pupils again to-day show a variable condition at different times. Five relaxed motions, vomited once, much sneezing. 45 grains of chloral were given at night, but brought up immediately.

April 2.—No sleep, two relaxed motions, vomited three times, pains in the stomach, burning of the feet, sneezing. Patient feels very prostrate. Seven relaxed motions. *In the morning right pupil more dilated, in the afternoon more contracted than the left.* Patient got up for several hours. 45 grains of chloral.

April 3.—Two hours' sleep altogether, relaxed motion, vomited once ; great restlessness, burning of the feet, pains in the calves and severe pains in the stomach. Patient also during the day is very restless, cannot remain quiet in any position, feels pain in the sacral region, has stomach- and headache. Face red. *Pupils equally contracted. There is fluttering when reading.*

April 4.—One and a half hours' sleep, restless, great prostration. Pulse 64, full, regular. Appetite moderate ; five relaxed motions. At 6 P.M. a warm bath is given. Sneezing.

April 5.—No sleep ; epigastric pain, restlessness, two relaxed motions ; less restlessness during the day, now and then shivering or feeling of heat. Patient still is very weak, has to take hold of the walls when walking. Pupils equal. 45 grains of chloral at night.

April 6.—Three and a half hours' sleep altogether ; restless ; epigastric pain ; burning of the feet. Patient felt weak during the day ; much perspiration. Appetite good. Right pupil somewhat more dilated than left. 30 grains of chloral.

April 7.—Four hours' sleep. Restless in the day. Patient was out in the garden. Appetite good, one opening of the bowels. *Right pupil more dilated than left* ; 30 grains of chloral. General condition good.

April 9.—Has slept little to-day ; there is again more restlessness in the limbs. Epigastric pains, weakness. Pupils equal.

April 14.—Has hardly slept at all ; feels pretty well throughout the day. Appetite good. Still asks for morphia now and then. Restless in the evening.

April 16.—Five hours' sleep without chloral ; two relaxed motions. Patient still feels weak and knocked up. Swimming before the eyes when reading.

April 21.—Has had hardly any sleep on account of intense pain in the legs and hypochondriac regions, which, although less severe, lasts throughout the day. 30 grains of chloral. *Left pupil larger than right.*

April 28.—The menstrual discharge has come on. Patient left the Institution May 6, 1876.

The examination of the urine gave the following results :— Quantity as usual, specific gravity 1·007 to 1·012. The urine reduced alkaline solution of sulphate of copper, turned the polarized light towards the left and contained large quantities of albumen. The microscopic examination, during the first fortnight of her staying with us, showed gelatinous cylinders and white corpuscles of blood; five weeks afterwards there were yet only slight traces of albumen. According to a communication of *Dr. Vorman,* at present medical director of the hospital to which sister M. belongs, the albumen had entirely disappeared after a further period of three weeks. Patient has had no relapse.

VI. Albuminuria during the period of abstinence.

B. S., medical practitioner, 46 years of age, married, was in 1874 afflicted with acute articular rheumatism, which compelled him to use morphia injections. After the disease had left, he stopped the drug, but resorted to it again on account of worry, injecting up to the time of his admission into the Institution on the average 8 grains per day, the highest dose being 16 grains. The result of the habitual use of the drug was *emaciation, loss of appetite, disposition to sweat, giddiness, loss of sleep ;* sexual power gone for a few hours after the use of each injection. Several months ago patient was afflicted with attacks of chill, heat and perspiration, principally at night.

Present state.—Patient is small and stout. Muscles and subcutaneous fatty layer pretty well developed. The internal organs according to examination are in a normal condition. On July 18, at night, patient had the last injection.

July 19.—Patient has had hardly any sleep during the night, moving about frequently, yawning, moaning, feeling as if he was going to die. Complains of epigastric pain, screams ; restlessness in the legs ; prostration ; little appetite. Intense craving for morphia. Pulse irregular, strong. At 9.30 P.M. 30 grains of chloral.

July 20.—Patient has slept for one hour and a half. There was epigastric pain, restlessness, sneezing and vomiting throughout the night. In the day time he had hyperæsthesia of the skin, sensibility of the eyes and ears to strong light and noise. Feeling of giddiness. There is excessive tendency for vomiting. Pulse 72.

July 21.—No sleep, patient remains quietly in bed ; had five relaxed motions in the night. Pupils equally wide. Throughout the day an uncomfortable feeling is predominant. Patient gets up for three hours. At 10 P.M. 30 grains of chloral in capsules are given.

July 22.—Patient has slept altogether for two hours, with many interruptions. During the day he feels better than hitherto. The diarrhœa, sneezing, and yawning, have not yet left him. Appetite poor.

July 25.—Patient during the last few nights has slept on the average from five to six hours. General condition a little better. Sneezing, yawning, and diarrhœa still occur several times in the day. Patient walked about in the garden for several hours.

July 27.—During the last two nights, patient after taking 45 grains of chloral each night, slept for five hours without interruption. He still feels very prostrate and restless ; complains of pain in the region of the stomach ; sneezing.

August 2.—Patient's appetite has returned again. Bowels regular. He feels well in himself. Sleep good.

August 10.—All the bodily functions are in a normal condition. Sleep good.

August 14.—Patient leaves the Institution and has had no relapse.

Examination of the urine : quantity moderate. Specific gravity from 1·026 to 1·035. In consequence of the high gravity of the urine, all re-agents for the detection of sugar were tried, but with a negative result. Albumen was distinctly discernible, but in small quantity ; no morphotic elements.

It is worth noticing in this case that the albumen, after having disappeared for several days, was present again for a short time. Four weeks after, when patient left the Institution, the urine did not contain any albumen.

VII. Albuminuria during the Period of Abstinence.

Mr. N., a merchant, a patient of Dr. Bartels, of Berlin, suffering from a hereditary predisposition to sick headache, was in the secondary stage of syphilis, and became afflicted with morbid

craving for morphia for the last four years through suffering from
iritis syphilitica, accompanied by headache. Highest daily dose
16 to 24 grains of morphia. In consequence of the injections
there was loss of appetite, constipation, shivering, perspiration,
impotence.

The patient, admitted into the Institution on May 19, 1876, is
strongly built and well nourished. Heart and lungs in a normal
state. Pulse 72, regular, somewhat tiny. Enlargement of some
of the cervical glands. Papulous eruption on the head. A swelling of the bone on the forehead is at times noticeable, and is said
to have appeared a week previously. Defluvium capillitii. *Left
pupil more contracted than right*, both reacting well. Urine contains no albumen.

On May 20 at 1 P.M. the last injection of 2 grains of morphia
was administered.

May 21.—Patient has slept until the morning, and has perspired a little. *Different condition of the pupils observable;* little
headache. Frequent shivering; epigastric pain; face red. In
the afternoon still gently perspiring, frequent paroxysms of sneezing, increased lachrymal secretion, one relaxed motion, vomited
twice.

May 22.—Has hardly slept at all. In the morning very weak.
Nausea; pulse 57, irregular, full. The epigastric pain increases
during the morning as well as the prostration; the former was
successfully relieved by the application of warm compresses to the
epigastrium. Five relaxed motions, vomited four times during
the day. 45 grains of chloral at night. *The urine shows traces of
albumen.*

May 23.—Patient has slept for two hours. Little pain in the
stomach. From 4 A.M. he becomes restless, moving about in bed;
vomited twice during the night. Pulse 78, regular. During daytime prostration, languid pains in the stomach, nausea, sickness,
feels as if the feet were dead; frequent sneezing. Three relaxed
motions, vomited once. *Urine contains albumen.*

May 24.—After 45 grains of chloral patient slept for about
five hours with interruptions. Appetite begins to return. One
relaxed motion. *Urine contains albumen.* 45 grains of chloral at
night.

May 25.—Very frequent sneezing. *Urine still becomes somewhat cloudy after being boiled and acetic acid added.*

May 27.—45 grains of chloral at night. Patient has slept with very little interruption. *No albumen in the urine.*

On the tenth day treatment with ointment of mercury was commenced. The genital powers showed renewed activity by the occurrence of erections ; the urine contained albumen only until the cessation of the symptoms of abstinence, which proved that the albuminuria could not be caused by the syphilis.

On June 27 patient leaves the Institution after having been treated with the ointment of mercury for four weeks.

He has not had a relapse.

EXPERIMENTS ON ANIMALS.

Date	Time	Dose of Morphia (Injected)	Albumen in the Urine	Morphia in the Urine
Small Young Rabbit.				
1876		Grains		
August 10	—	—	None	—
,, 11	9 A.M.	$1\frac{1}{2}$	—	—
,, 11	7 P.M.	$1\frac{1}{2}$	—	—
,, 12	—	—	Traceable	Traceable
,, 13	—	—	Distinctly discernible	,,
,, 14	—	—	Traceable	,,
,, 15	—	—	Slight trace	None
,, 16	—	—	Gone	—
,, 17	9 A.M.	$\frac{1}{2}$	—	—
,, 17	7 P.M.	$\frac{1}{2}$	—	Traceable
,, 18	9 A.M.	$\frac{1}{2}$	In large quantity	,,
,, 18	7 P.M.	$\frac{1}{2}$	—	,,
,, 19	9 A.M.	$\frac{1}{2}$	Traceable	,,
,, 20	—	—	,,	,,
,, 21	—	—	Only traces	,,
22	—	—	None	,,
23	—	—	—	None
Small Rabbit.				
August 11	9 A.M.	$1\frac{1}{2}$	—	—
,, 11	7 P.M.	$1\frac{1}{2}$	—	—
,, 12	7 P.M.		Traceable	Traceable
13	—	—	Large quantity	,,
14	—	—	,,	None
15	—	—	Traces	,,

Date	Time	Dose of Morphia (Injected)	Albumen in the urine	Morphia in the urine
1876		Grains		
August 16	—	—	None	None
,, 17	9 A.M.	$\frac{1}{2}$	—	—
,, 17	7 P.M.	$\frac{1}{2}$	—	Traceable
,, 18	9 A.M.	$\frac{1}{2}$	—	,,
,, 18	7 P.M.	$\frac{1}{2}$	Distinctly dis-cernible	,,
,, 19	—	—	Traceable	,,
,, 20	—	—	,,	,,
,, 21	—	—	,,	None
,, 22	—	—	Traces	,,
,, 23	—	—	Gone	,,
,, 25	7 P.M.	$\frac{1}{6}$	—	—
,, 26	—	—	Traces	Traceable
,, 27	7 P.M.	$\frac{1}{12}$	—	—
,, 28	—	—	None	Traceable
,, 29	7 P.M.	$\frac{1}{6}$	—	—
,, 30	—	—	Traceable	Traceable
,, 31	—	—	Gone	Gone

Middle-sized Rabbit.

Date	Time	Dose of Morphia (Injected)	Albumen in the urine	Morphia in the urine
September 11	7 P.M.	$\frac{1}{20}$	—	—
,, 12	—	—	None	None
,, 12	7 P.M.	$\frac{1}{10}$	,,	—
,, 13	—	—	,,	Distinctly dis-cernible
,, 13	7 P.M.	$\frac{1}{7}$	—	—
,, 14	—	—	None	Distinctly dis-cernible
,, 14	7 P.M.	$\frac{1}{5}$	—	—
,, 15	—	—	None	Distinctly dis-cernible
,, 15	7 P.M.	$\frac{1}{4}$	—	—
,, 16	—	—	None	Distinctly dis-cernible
,, 16	7 P.M.	$\frac{1}{4}$	—	—
,, 17	—	—	None	Distinctly dis-cernible
,, 17	7 P.M.	$\frac{1}{3}$	—	—
,, 18	—	—	None	Distinctly dis-cernible
,, 18	7 P.M.	$\frac{2}{5}$	—	—
,, 19	—	—	None	Distinctly dis-cernible
,, 19	7 P.M.	$\frac{7}{15}$	—	—
,, 20	—	—	Traces	Distinctly dis-cernible

Date	Time	Dose of Morphia (Injected)	Albumen in the Urine	Morphia in the Urine
1876 September 20	7 P.M.	Grains $\frac{1}{2}$	—	—
,, 21	—	—	Traces	Distinctly discernible
,, 21	7 P.M.	$\frac{1}{2}$	—	—
,, 22	—	—	Great quantity	Distinctly discernible
,, 22	7 P.M.	$\frac{7}{12}$	—	—
,, 23	—	—	Distinctly discernible	Distinctly discernible
24	—	Discontinued	Ditto	Ditto
25	—	—	Ditto	Ditto
,, 26	—	—	Traces	Gone
,, 27	—	—	,,	—
,, 28	—	—	,,	—
,, 29	—	—	,,	—
October 3	—	—	Gone	—
,, 4	—	—	,,	—
,, 5	—	—	,,	—

Large Rabbit.

Date	Time	Dose of Morphia (Injected)	Albumen in the Urine	Morphia in the Urine
October 12	—	—	None	None
,, 12	2.25 P.M.	$\frac{2}{3}$	—	,,
,, 13	—	—	—	—
,, 13	1.30 P.M.	$\frac{1}{3}$	—	—
,, 14	—	—	—	Traceable
,, 14	8.30 A.M.	$\frac{1}{3}$	—	,,
,, 14	1.30 P.M.	$\frac{5}{6}$	Distinctly discernible	,,
,, 15	—	—	Ditto	,,
,, 15	1.30 P.M.	$\frac{2}{3}$	—	,,
,, 16	—	—	Traceable	,,
,, 16	8 P.M.	$\frac{3}{4}$	—	,,
,, 17	—	—	Distinctly traceable	,,
,, 17	8 P.M.	1	—	—
,, 18	—	—	Traceable	,,
,, 19	—	—	Distinctly traceable	,,
20	—	—	Traceable	None
21	—	—	Traces	,,
22	—	—	,,	,,
23	—	—	—	,,
24	—	—	Gone	,,

H

Date	Time	Dose of Morphia (Injected)	Albumen in the Urine	Morphia in the Urine

Middle-sized Rabbit.

Date	Time	Dose of Morphia (Injected) Grains	Albumen in the Urine	Morphia in the Urine
1876 October 12	—	—	None	—
,, 12	2.25 P.M.	$\frac{1}{3}$	—	None
,, 13	—	—	None	Traceable
,, 13	1.30 P.M.	$\frac{1}{2}$	—	,,
,, 14	—	—	Traceable	,,
,, 14	—	—	—	,,
,, 15	—	—	Distinct traces	None
,, 15	—	—	—	,,
,, 16	—	—	Traces	,,
,, 16	—	—	—	,,
,, 17	8 A.M.	$1\frac{1}{3}$	—	,,
,, 17	Afternoon	—	Traceable	Traceable
,, 18	—	—	,,	,.
,, 19	—	—	,,	
,, 20	—	—	Traces	None
,, 21	—	—	,,	,,
,, 22	—	—	Gone	,,
,, 23	—	—	—	,,
,, 24	—	—	—	,,

Middle-sized Female Dog.

Date	Time	Dose of Morphia (Injected)	Albumen in the Urine	Morphia in the Urine
October 10	—	—	None	
,, 11	—	—	—	
,, 12	2.25 P.M.	$\frac{1}{6}$	—	
,, 12	8 P.M.	$\frac{1}{3}$	—	
,, 13	1.30 P.M.	$\frac{2}{3}$	—	
,, 14	8.30 ,,	$\frac{1}{3}$	—	
,, 14	1.30 ,,	$\frac{1}{3}$	—	
,, 15	—	—	Distinctly traceable	
,, 15	1.30 P.M.	I	—	
,, 16	—	—	Distinctly traceable	
,, 16	8 A.M.	$1\frac{1}{3}$	—	
,, 17	—	—	In large quantities	
,, 17	8 A.M.	$1\frac{1}{2}$	—	
,, 18	—	—	In large quantities	
,, 18	—	—	—	
,, 19	—	—	Distinctly discernible	
,, 20	—	—	Traceable	
,, 21	—	—	Traces	
,, 22	—	—	—	
,, 23	—	—	Gone	
,, 24	—	—	,,	

Date	Time	Dose of Morphia (Injected)	Albumen in the Urine	Morphia in the Urine
			Small Dog.	
1876 October 13	—	Grains —	None	
„ 13	1 P.M.	1	—	
„ 14	—	—	Traceable	
„ 14	8.45 A.M.	$1\frac{1}{3}$	—	
„ 14	1.30 P.M.	$1\frac{1}{2}$	Traceable	
„ 15	—	—	„	
„ 18	—	—	None	

A middle-sized dog, whose urine, according to several days' examination, contained no albumen, was treated with an injection of 4 grains of morphia on the morning of October 26.

The visible effects of the injection were : complete paralysis of the hind legs, and consequent inability to stand up ; salivation and somnolence ; forty-eight hours after the urine already contained albumen, the latter increasing in quantity until November 2, afterwards gradually disappearing. The urine reduced alkaline solution of sulfate of copper without, however, turning the polarised light.

A small dog was for nine days injected with $2\frac{2}{3}$ grains of morphia per day. On the third day albumen was found in the urine, which continued in the same quantity till the day of his death, showing all the characteristic reactions.

A large female dog was treated for seven days with daily injections of 3 grains of morphia. The urine, which was normal previously, contained pretty large quantities of albumen by the third day : on the fifth day it contained blood, which continued till the sixth. Apart from red blood-corpuscles, the microscopic examination showed some corpuscles of pus.

On the seventh day the animal died. The post-mortem examination, performed at once, showed both kidneys highly congested. The bladder, on its outer surface, showed small varicose veins, which also completely covered its inner coating.

In order to explain this albuminuria[1] we are, through the want of positive pathological facts, confined to hypotheses, of which the three following may be considered :—

The appearance of albumen may be caused :

(1.) By the action of morphia on the central organ, which has a relation to albumen.

(2.) By the concurrence of anomalies in the normal pressure of the blood, causing at last intra-renal disorders.[2]

(3.) By paralysis of the nerves which surround the arteria renalis. This paralysis would have the same effect as the separation by knife of the nerves encircling the renal artery, after doing which von Wittich found albumen in the urine.

It is very probable that the origin of the albuminuria is due to the varying pressure of the blood, which, according to experience, is caused by the action of morphia.

These fluctuations would also explain the intermittent occurrence of the albuminuria in the different stages of morbid craving for morphia, i. e., its sporadic appearance during the use of the drug, as well as its appearance on the first and on the eighth day following the abstinence. Those cases, showing a continuous presence of albumen during all the three stages of morbid craving for morphia, must be attributed to a paralysis of the nerves of the renal artery.

---

[1] Munk und Leyden, ' Die acute Phosphorvergiftung,' 1865.
[2] Beneke, ' Pathologie des Stoffwechsels,' 1874, p. 222.

Regarding the influence of morphia on the medulla oblongata, it seems that it only becomes affected by fatal doses. This supposition gained strength by the following experiments, in which I found sugar, besides the albumen. The occurrence of sugar in the human body caused by a poisonous dose I had occasion to verify some time previously. I shall, for the sake of comparison, relate this case before proceeding to the various experiments on animals.

CASE.

Acute Morphia Poisoning.

On June 11, 1875, a lady was by mistake subjected to an injection of 5 grains of morphia from a solution containing 25% of the drug. It at once caused severe pain at the place of injection and oppressive symptoms of the utmost gravity.

Twenty minutes later I found her with a dark red face and suffering from giddiness and drowsiness, the carotides beating intensely, the pupils being contracted to a minimum. Pulse 92, respiration 24. I made an injection of one-fortieth of a grain of atropia, repeating it twice at short intervals, as the pupils did not react. At last they began to dilate, the drowsiness and somnolence however increasing; the speech became slow, difficult, and un-intelligible, the face of a dark red, the eyes bright.

Patient had some black coffee given, an ice-bag was applied to the head and leeches to both process. mastoid. and the nasal mucous membrane, but apparently without success. To keep her from falling asleep, a tepid bath with cold douche was given, and the patient made to walk about, supported by two persons. The respiration having sunk to four inspirations in the minute, I fara-dised the nerv. phrenicus. Patient neither noticed anyone talking to her, nor could be roused by stimulants; had to be put to bed, and sank into a deep sleep four hours after the poisoning had occurred. After the lapse of half an hour, the respiration having sunk to three per minute, it was again necessary to resort to Faradisation.

The patient by this means woke up, smiling pleasantly; her face became paler, the pupils larger; she, however, immediately fell asleep again. The sleep this time was a short one, as she began to vomit severely every half-hour; a state of delirium followed, which allowed the patient to rest for a short time only. The respiration had increased to six per minute.

About twelve hours after the poisoning the severe bodily symptoms began to abate, patient again completely recovering her senses. Patient for a fortnight after the mishap remained in a weak condition, felt giddy, and was unable to walk or to think quickly.

On the second day the urine, drawn off in the night by the catheter, was examined; showing a light blue colour when mixed with a solution of caustic soda and sulfate of copper. After being heated the oxyhydrate of copper in solution was reduced to oxydulate of copper, the addition of alkali and bismuth producing a black colour when heated. The polarised light was turned towards the right for two or three fractional parts of the Soleil-Ventzke apparatus. Several days afterwards the pathological alterations of the urine had disappeared.

EXPERIMENTS ON ANIMALS.

I.

A large rabbit was given $4\frac{1}{2}$ grains of morphia at 4 o'clock. Immediate somnolence. Reaction of the bulbi diminished; death at 6 o'clock.

Post-mortem Examination three hours after.—On pressing the abdomen 96 cubic centimetres of a light yellow urine passed out of the bladder, showing a slight flaky sediment. Specific gravity, 1·019. The urine shows the following condition:—

1. It precipitated a large quantity of red oxydulate of copper out of Fehling's solution.

2. It reduced pernitrate of bismuth.

3. With yeast active alcoholic fermentation was produced in it.

4. It turned the polarised light for four fractional parts of the Soleil-Ventzke apparatus.

5. It changed its colour when boiled with a solution of caustic soda.

6. On applying Trommer's test, it showed great reduction of colour without however precipitating red oxydulate of copper.

7. It contained traces of albumen.

II.

A large rabbit was given 7 grains of morphia at 5 P.M.   It died in three quarters of an hour.

Post-mortem Examination two hours afterwards.— The urine forced out by pressure of the abdomen showed the following condition :—

1. It reduced alkaline solution of sulfate of copper, precipitating red oxydulate of copper.

2. The same with Fehling's solution.

3. After adding yeast and exposing it to a temperature of 40° R. (104° F.), it evolved carbonic acid gas after a short time.

4. It reduced pernitrate of bismuth.

5. Turns polarised light towards the right.

6. It contains albumen in clearly perceptible quantity.

On dissection, the corticalis of the kidneys is of a dark red colour. Substance of the liver flabby, can be crushed with a slight pressure of the finger. Stomach and intestines very full. The left ventricle feels extremely hard, the right is soft and flabby. Both contain coagulated blood.

III.

A large rabbit is treated at 9.30 with an injection of 7 grains of morphia under the skin of the back.   Died half an hour afterwards.

Post-mortem Examination two hours afterwards.— The urine evacuated from the bladder (quantity, about 106 cubic centimetres) did not contain any sugar, but slight quantities of albumen. The internal organs show no abnormal condition. The rigidity, showing itself at the moment of dying, was worthy of notice.

IV.

A middle-sized rabbit had at 3 P.M. 5 grains of morphia injected under the skin of the back. The animal continued to live. The urine passed during the night (54 cubic centimetres) contained no albumen, but showed all the reactions for sugar in a most distinct manner.

1. The examination with Fehling's solution showed a quantity of sugar, 0·75 per cent.

2. The fermentation of the urine, when mixed with yeast, was very brisk.

3. The trial with bismuth, Trommer's solution, and caustic soda, gave a positive result.

4. The polarised light is turned towards the right.

The following day (November 21) the animal was fed with cabbage leaves only. The urine (96 cubic centimetres) contained sugar, although in smaller quantity than the day before.

On November 22, at 11 A.M., 5 grains of morphia were again injected into the animal's skin. Deep somnolence. Died in the night.

Post-mortem Examination in the afternoon of November 23.—The bladder contains about 15 cubic centimetres of urine, not giving any reactions when tested for sugar.

V.

A large rabbit was fastened down to a board at 11.30 A.M., and tracheotomy was performed.

At 11.45, 7 grains of morphia were injected under the skin of the abdomen.

At 12 A.M., dyspnœa coming on, artificial respiration was resorted to.

At 12.45 P.M., 1 grain of morphia was given to the animal.

At 2.45 P.M., artificial respiration was stopped.

By removing the canula, the animal died.

The urine removed from the bladder showed *quantities of sugar by all reactions* (the light turned towards the right, reduction of *Fehling's* and *Trommer's* solution). Traces of albumen present.

VI.

Middle-sized rabbit.—1 grain of morphia was given at 2.12 P.M.

At 3.10 P.M. the animal died under opisthotonus.

The urine taken from the bladder (about 35 cubic centimetres) gives a clear precipitate of oxydulate of copper with *Fehling's*, as well as with *Trommer's*, solution. Pernitrate of bismuth is reduced. Polarised light is turned towards the right. Albuminous dulness plainly perceptible on the addition of nitric acid.

VII.

A **large rabbit** is injected at 8 A.M. with 1 grain of morphia.

At 8.34 A.M. the animal died in convulsions.

About 74 cubic centimetres of urine are taken from the completely filled bladder. It contained sugar, which could be proved as such by all the respective reactions.

There were only traces of albumen.

VIII.

A **middle-sized female dog** was treated with daily injections of 2 grains of morphia for twenty-three days. On the fourth day after its administration the urine contained albumen.

After having stopped the drug for a week, the animal at 9 A.M. was injected with 15 grains of morphia.

It continued to live. Forty-eight hours afterwards urine was passed, *containing large quantities of sugar, which was proved by the turning of the polarised light towards the right, by fermentation, and by Fehling's and Trommer's reaction.*

The urine passed three days afterwards was *perfectly devoid of sugar.* On the fourth day, an injection of 25 grains of morphia was made. The urine passed two days after this poisoning (54 cubic centimetres) answered to all reactions for sugar (turning the light towards the right, fermentation, reduction of oxide of copper, etc.).

IX.

A **large dog** was injected with 24 grains of morphia. Urine was not passed till one and a-half days afterwards. It was proved to contain a substance capable of strong power of reduction, which, however, could not be identified with sugar.[1] The animal continued to live. The respective substance again disappeared. The urine passed after a further injection of 40 grains of morphia

[1] Quincke, ' Berl. Klin. Wochenschrift,' 1876, No. 38.

reduced the alkaline solution of sulfate of copper and of bis
muth, turned dark brown when boiled with solution of caustic
soda ; did not turn the light. The quantitative analysis of a
fractional part of the urine for morphia showed the presence of
about 15 grains in the whole quantity collected for examination.

This diabetes, following a fatal dose of morphia,
is in accordance with the already known glycosuria
following fatal poisoning with curare,[1] oxide of
carbon,[2] chloral[3], and chloroform; it has its origin,
probably, in the medulla oblongata, inasmuch as the
latter causes the first severe symptoms after the
poisoning.

The presence of sugar in the urine after the administration of poisonous doses of morphia, which,
according to the above-mentioned case relating to
the human body, and according to the results of the
experiments on animals, must be considered as of
frequent occurrence, will have a legal importance
henceforth. The absence of sugar in the urine, in a
case of suspected poisoning by morphia, would, at
least, render it doubtful as to whether the death was
caused by morphia. The case would be decided if,
although the urine showed a negative condition, the
quantitative analysis should show a quantity of
morphia sufficient to prove fatal, according to
experience.

---

[1] Dock, 'Pflueger's Archiv,' v., 571 ; and Winogradoff, 'Virchow's
Archiv,' xxvii., p. 533.

[2] Kühne, 'Physiolog. Chemie,' 1868, p. 521.

[3] Levinstein, 'Berlin. Klin. Wochenschrift,' 1876, No. 27.

PROGRESS OF THE DISEASE.

The progress of morbid craving for morphia, until it becomes a severe illness, is generally slow, and is subject to many fluctuations.

Some individuals are able to take large doses of morphia (up to 15 grains) for many years without any visible symptoms, while, with others, small doses will, after a few months, bring on loss of appetite and a changeable condition of mind, accompanied by neuralgic complaints, loss of sleep, etc.

The small quantity of food taken soon gives rise to general disorders, showing themselves as bodily weakness, and as pathological alterations in the different nervous regions. For a long time, however, all these morbid conditions will be kept in check by the continuous administration of the drug.

Like alcoholic intoxication, the morbid symptoms of our disease have clear intermissions, during which time, although the use of morphia is continued (mostly in diminished doses), all the disorders are disappearing. Changes in the habitual way of living, in social position, important affairs acting upon the mind, will greatly contribute towards such occurrences.

But this seeming improvement only lasts for a short time, hardly for a few months. Soon the morbid disorders will increase through the administration of the previous larger doses of morphia, and gradually all the various symptoms of the disease in question will become permanent.

The ultimate result of morbid craving for morphia, if no cure is effected, is a state of prostration, leading to marasmus and death.

PROGNOSIS.

The prognosis is favourable with regard to the abstinence, dubious with respect to the relapses. These latter are dependent on each individual constitution, on the customs, the mode of life and the state of health of the respective patients : they are less to be dreaded in energetic natures, sound in body and mind and possessing the power of resistance.   There is more hope for an absolute cure for those who get accustomed to the injections of morphia during the course of an acute disease, than for cases where the drug was resorted to on account of neuro- and psychopathic derangements, and chronical diseases.

The prognosis is less favourable if the patients have a craving for alcoholic beverages.   The relapses occur most readily immediately after the period of abstinence, their frequency being in a reverse relation to the duration of this abstinence from morphia.

People suffering from morbid craving for morphia, and using smaller doses of the drug, generally have relapses less frequently than those using larger doses; but this, as aforesaid, is dependent on the individual constitution. I have seen people remain free from relapse although injecting 25 to 30 grains of morphia daily. The relapse may be caused already by slight bodily disturbance, but principally by circumstances affecting the mind, such as domestic troubles, distress, and worry.

The administration of injections of morphia to patients who have been cured of morbid craving for morphia is to be carefully avoided, and must not be recommended, as otherwise they would be most certainly led back to their previous unhappy state. *One injection administered to a person who has been cured of morbid craving for morphia, will prove sufficient to vanquish the power of resistance against the craving for morphia successfully kept up for months together.*

TREATMENT.

The chief principle in the treatment of morbid craving for morphia is the deprivation of the drug, the sudden process being preferable to the slow deprivation.

Several authors[1] have adopted the slow deprivation, being of opinion that the sudden withdrawal in cases where the patients have for years past been accustomed to large doses of morphia is not advisable, and is attended with danger on account of the

---

[1] *Lähr*, Fiedler l. c. *Leidesdorff.* 'Die Morphiumsucht,' *Wiener Medic. Wochenschrift*, 1876, No. 25.

severe symptoms of reaction. The cases mentioned in this work are conclusive evidence that these suppositions are not justified, and that bad results only follow, if the proper precautions are omitted which are required in the treatment of morbid craving for morphia.

The reasons which have induced me to resort to the sudden deprivation, and to make use of it in the treatment,[1] are as follow :—the complaints following upon every deprivation of the morphia are not of so violent a form when the drug is slowly withdrawn, but they continue for a longer period of time. After the sudden deprivation the patients generally overcome the severest symptoms in two or three days, while the others suffer for weeks together, not escaping any of the many symptoms following the abstinence.

The human organisation, as we know from surgery, midwifery, etc., will, in general, submit more easily to sudden and energetic treatment, even when acting powerfully, than to a milder influence. The gradual deprivation, requiring a long time, excites the physical and moral powers to a greater extent, because every dose smaller than the previous day's quantity will produce new symptoms of reaction. The constant mental anxiety in which these patients live, while expecting a smaller dose on the following

---

[1] 'Die Morphiumsucht,' *Berl. Klin. Wochenschr.*, 1875, No. 48 ; 'Zur Pathologie der acuten Morphium- und Chloralvergiftung,' *Ibid.*, 1876, No. 27. See also Richter, 'Berl. Klin. Wochenschr.,' 1876, No. 28.

day, makes them fretful and irritable,—their intention of submitting till the end of the cure and their
energy begin to decline, and they try to evade the
treatment. They set up intrigues against the
officials and nurses ; they simulate morbid appearances, in order to cause the pity of their relations
and friends ; they lose confidence in themselves and
in their doctor, whose full and absolute authority is
indispensable for the successful treatment of abstinence.

In cases of sudden deprivation, on the contrary,
the confidence in the medical adviser is strengthened
in consequence of the short duration of the severe
symptoms, and the improvement, already experienced
after a few days ; the patients take courage, look
forward to their complete recovery, and submit with
patience and resignation to the few days of suffering.

To treat morbid craving for morphia with
success, it is necessary to decide the principal question, namely, whether each individual patient does,
or does not, suffer from pathological complaints or
chronic disorders requiring narcotics for their relief.
If he does, it is only necessary for the doctor to
deprive the patient of the morphia *syringe* and to
inject personally, if his time permits of so doing, a
dose which he thinks sufficient, or else to give the
narcotic internally.

Furthermore, we exclude from the treatment all
patients weak or exhausted through bodily or mental
affliction. It is all the same whether the pros-

tration is caused by night duty, distress, illness, childbed, want of proper food, flooding, etc.; only those conditions of weakness following upon the poisoning with morphia constitute no counterindication, as they disappear in consequence of the deprivation. Only such individuals, therefore, are suited for the treatment who have continued the injections while in perfect health, the former morbid appearances for which they at first administered them having disappeared.

For the sake of avoiding trouble during the treatment of people afflicted with morbid craving for morphia, it is necessary to distinctly tell the patients that, for the first week of the treatment, they would have to forego the exercise of their own free will and submit, without opposition, to the orders of the medical attendant. They are patients who have to get rid of a passion which has command over them; and as morbid craving for morphia, like other passions, debases men, the variable disposition of their character, apart from the other conditions of bodily weakness, is not to be lost sight of. This debasement mainly shows itself as a tendency for untruthfulness. Educated, intelligent, and hitherto respectable ladies and gentlemen will so far forget themselves as to lie wilfully. Hardly any person suffering from morbid craving for morphia is able truthfully to state the daily quantity of morphia used, and the hour when he last injected morphia. It is imperative that this weakness should be taken

into account, and consequently the statements of the
patients are not to be trusted; but, on the other
hand, it is not advisable to induce them to this state
of untruthfulness, arising from internal causes, by
pressing them with questions. It is well to treat
them like people under age, of course not deviating
from the usage of society, and to protect them from
temptations by keeping a watch on them. As soon
as the patient has consented to give up his personal
liberty, and the treatment is about to commence, he
is to be shown into the rooms set apart for him for a
period of eight to fourteen days, all opportunities for
attempting suicide having been removed from them.
Doors and windows must not move on hinges, but
in pivots; must have neither handles, nor bolts or
keys, being so constructed that the patients can
neither open nor shut them. Hooks for looking
glasses, for clothes and curtains must be removed.
The bedroom, for the sake of control, is to have only
the most necessary furniture: a bed, devoid of
protruding bedposts, a couch, an open washstand,
a table furnished with alcoholic stimulants (champagne, port wine, brandy), ice in small pieces, and a
tea urn with the necessary implements. In the
room which is to serve as a residence for the medical
attendant for the first three days, the following drugs
are to be kept under lock and key :—a solution of
morphia of 2 per cent., chloroform, æther, ammonia,
liq. ammon. anis.; mustard, an ice bag, and an elec-

tric induction apparatus.   A bath-room may adjoin
these two apartments.   During the first four or five
days of the abstinence, the patient must be constantly watched by two female nurses.   Male attendants are of no use in cases of morbid craving for
morphia, as they are generally more accessible to
bribing, and are less to be relied upon and less
capable of self-sacrifice.   They are, however, wanted
for the coarser manipulations, for attending to the
bath of male patients, and may then be admitted
under supervision.

The treatment is more agreeable for the patient
and easier for the medical attendant, if the first nurse
is an educated person, well acquainted with the requirements and wants of the higher classes.   The
nurses must be tested as to their energy and per-
severance ; we can warmly recommend deaconesses
for private nursing, on account of their conscien-
tiousness and fidelity.

During the first four or five days, the nurses
must be changed every twelve hours, as the service
requires mental and physical ability, and is very
fatiguing.

Immediately after admission the patient has to
take a warm bath ; during the time of taking it a
confidential person has to search all his things for
morphia, which, notwithstanding the patient's assur-
ances to the contrary, is sometimes concealed in
the most ingenious manner.   Almost all persons
entering upon a treatment for the sake of abstinence

from morphia are carrying morphia and a syringe with them.

Only after we have done this can we commence the treatment with the assurance of not being deluded.

The first symptoms of the abstinence, showing themselves in weak persons after three or four hours, in stronger people frequently as late as fifteen hours, after the last injection of morphia, such as uncomfortable feeling, languid pain in the limbs, yawning, sneezing, slight chill, are no objects for treatment ; severe shivering necessitates going to bed, in order to become warm, which, on account of the depressed state of mind. is readily agreed to by the patients.

Against the usually prevalent headache, cold water and iced compresses, æther dropped on the forehead, or on the skull, may be recommended ; against the severe griping pains in the epigastric region, compresses, moistened with chloroform, may be applied. Abdominal pains occurring seldom, but being very distressing, are relieved by mustard plasters and hot cataplasms ; on account of their simplicity we use the ' Cataplasmes Instantanés.'

Nausea and vomiting, as well as the dyspepsia, lasting for several days, are successfully treated by a solution of bicarbonate of soda, with tinct. nuc. vomic. and ol. menth. pip. Should the vomiting become more frequent, at first ice pills, mustard plasters on the epigastrium, or instead of the latter a local application of chloroform, may be resorted to.

In case, however, it should repeat itself twenty or thirty times in the twenty-four hours, thus threatening to exhaust the patient's strength, 1 to 3 tablespoonfuls of a solution of morphia (1 grain in 6 ounces) may be given.

Should the patient refuse to take food on account of the continuous vomiting, and should severe symptoms of prostration set in, nourishing injections into the rectum must be administered.

Diarrhœa, occurring regularly during the period of abstinence, is no object for treatment, as it mostly disappears of itself after a few days. Should it become of a severe character, however, or last longer than three or four days, warm water injections into the bowel (temp. 37° C., 98·6 F.) of 1 to 2 pints, repeated two or three times in the day, will prove of great benefit.

The *sleeplessness* will resist any treatment during the first three or four days, and is the symptom mostly complained of by the patients. Prolonged warm bathing will not be endured by the patients at this time, giving as it does at the most half-an-hour to one hour's sleep. Hydrate of chloral, per os, or per anum, does not either at this period create sleep, its use often being followed by great excitement. After the lapse of the first four days however it will agree with many patients, exercising in such instances its hypnotic effects.

The general debility and psychical depression of the first days will be successfully treated by warm baths, with cold douches of five minutes' duration. Do not allow yourself to be induced to abstain from giving them on account of any of the symptoms of abstinence, as all the patients suffering from the abuse of morphia, even if they have objected to the first bath, immediately begin to feel the comfort created by it, are refreshed afterwards, and impatiently long for a repetition. During the time of bathing, stimulants, such as champagne, port wine, beef tea, etc., may be given.

The greatest care during treatment is to be bestowed upon the diet, from the commencement of the withdrawal of the drug. During the first three days, food is only to be given in a fluid form; strong wines and, according to individual susceptibility, pure alcoholic liquors are to be resorted to. They are best given in the same manner as a medicine, every hour or two hours.

Many people have an intense craving for alcoholic beverages, others greatly objecting to them. The first-mentioned patients may be allowed to drink wine in unlimited quantities, without any ill effects, as by doing so they pass over the first days of the abstinence in a less distressing manner; should, however, there be reluctance and distaste for alcohol, a light milk diet (2 ounces of milk every hour, or two hours) may be ordered. This agrees well even with persons who are greatly troubled with vomiting.

With a diet regulated in such a manner from the

first day of the abstinence and persevered in as much as possible, even if the patient should oppose it, the severe collapse, occurring most certainly in cases of insufficient supply of food, will, undoubtedly, be prevented.

TREATMENT OF THE COLLAPSE.

The simple collapse will disappear under the above-mentioned dietetic regime, the severest forms, however, requiring an energetic and very attentive treatment.

It is advisable to guard against looking at every condition of exhaustion as collapse, and the same may be said of patients, especially females, possessing a great talent to simulate conditions resembling collapse ; but it is true, nevertheless, that a mistake made under such conditions is not of very great im portance, and would only have the disadvantage of prolonging the period of the treatment.

A medical man who does not lose his quiet composure when at the bedside, relying on the apparent facts and considering the intervening symptoms, will neither commit the above-mentioned mistake, nor be guilty of the irreparable fault of overlooking a severe collapse.

The symptoms of collapse requiring energetic action, are principally caused by the heart, less frequently by the brain, and only exceptionally by the lungs.

If the character of the pulse is changing, *i.e.*, the previously soft condition getting threadlike, sinking gradually or at once, after having become irregular, to one-third or a smaller fraction of its former normal frequency; if the patient's face is getting pale, the nose becoming pointed, and if the previous excitement suddenly is replaced by a quiet demeanour, or by fainting fits; if somnolence sets in accompanied by deep and slow respiration—an injection of ½ grain of morphia is to be administered at once as an indicatio vitalis. If within ten minutes the pulse and the general condition do not improve, the injection is to be repeated once or twice until the return of the normal condition is evident. At the same time the patient is to be kept awake by counter-irritation, smelling salts, cold compresses on the head, dropping æther on the skull, by talking loud to him and shaking him; and stimulants such as liq. ammon. anis., champagne, port wine, brandy, hot coffee or tea with rum, are to be given internally.

If on the dangerous symptoms subsiding, the patient falls asleep, the respiration and circulation must be watched.

Should the severe collapse return on the same or following day, the latter only occurring in quite exceptional cases, the same treatment must be resorted to.

Formerly I used to recommend injections of strychnia and liq. ammon. anisatus to overcome the dangerous weakness of the heart. Having, however, noticed the fact of its having been removed by an injection of morphia, and of the collapse generally being prevented by the regular and un-interrupted taking of food by the patient, I had no occasion to recur to the just mentioned remedies.

For the same reason the application of the in-duction current will be but rarely indicated, so as to gradually increase the faltering condition of the respiration in cases of sudden collapse.

It is worth noticing, that injections of morphia administered during the collapse, do not prolong the time of the severe symptoms of abstinence.

The delirium tremens chronicum does not require any particular treatment, as it disappears in the same manner as the albuminuria, double vision, etc., soon after the use of the drug is discontinued.

In cases of *delirium tremens acutum*, however, some precautions are to be observed. The patient, suffering from this kind of disease, must be lodged in a room, where he is prevented from doing himself any harm. No other furniture but a fixed couch, that cannot be taken to pieces, ought to be in the room. The windows must be constructed so that the patients cannot break them. The modern In-stitutions on this account are fitted with glass half-an-inch thick

If the patient is isolated, he will soon become quiet. If there is only moderate excitement, the warm bath, with the cold douche, will be found beneficial. Morphia injections during the delirium are not to be recommended. The short duration of acute delirium, the absence of severe collapse, render its occurrence of no importance whatever.

Impotence disappears at the end of the second week, the return of the often greatly increased sexual excitement requiring a milder diet, smaller quantities of wine, withdrawal of ardent spirits, and the daily use of a warm bath.

The *Amenorrhœa* ceases with the deprivation of morphia. The pains in the sacral region and the abdomen, lasting several days, and appearing before the return of the menstrual discharge, will be relieved by cataplasms, injections of tepid water, and warm baths.

One week after the commencement of the abstinence from morphia the most worrying symptoms, such as vomiting, diarrhœa, painful disorders on the part of the nervous system having already disappeared, and the patient having, to all appearance, entered into the convalescent state, we frequently notice the strange phenomenon (already observed years ago by Professor Westphal) of the whole group of symptoms of abstinence suddenly returning again. This renewed attack has a duration only of twenty-four to thirty-six hours, not influencing, however, the further progress. With or without this attack the loss of appetite is disappearing, and in its stead an increased desire for food is noticeable, which must be regulated according to each individual constitution. The principal symptoms still remaining behind are sleeplessness and general debility, and, if occurring altogether, albuminuria.

Although the vis medicatrix naturæ will gradu ally regulate all bodily disturbance, observable for a short time after the removal of the poison from the system, the three last mentioned conditions may be cured more rapidly by a proper after-treatment.

The sleeplessness, which is generally protracted up into the fourth week, is very distressing. Only in the case of the patient feeling exhausted, medicinal treatment may be adopted against it. On the other hand, it will be found advisable to create fatigue by ordering bodily activity, long continued walks, and warm baths at night.

The albuminuria, frequently lasting for several months, will disappear under the application of warm baths and a strengthening diet.

The general debility, especially in females, will not in many cases disappear till six or eight weeks after the withdrawal of the morphia. If the patients have the means, they may, in the fourth week, be sent to a mountainous district, or to the south of Europe, or to a cold water establishment, according to their strength and the season of the year. After wards they are not to be regarded any more as patients, and a full share of work, according to their social position, may be expected from them.

When speaking of the treatment of morbid craving for morphia, I had in my thoughts the sojourn of the patient at a hospital having a large

medical staff, and special medical attendants for each
day.   In private dwellings the treatment will only
be possible in exceptional cases, and with important
modifications.   In these cases the physician does
not always possess the necessary authority, as the
attendants and nurses are not in his, but in the
patient's, service.   The isolation of the patient from
his relations becomes impossible; the friends as well
as the patient will influence the treatment, and they
will deceive the doctor; finally, the medical supervision, which in this case must be divided among
several people, can only be realised under special
circumstances.

For the same reason the cold water establish
ments, as they are managed nowadays, may be
absolutely rejected with regard to the treatment of
morbid craving for morphia, as they do not possess
the proper hospital discipline; as the patients, who
have the right of keeping their own attendants, cannot be watched properly; and finally, as very often
there is not, and cannot be, the necessary medical
staff at their service.   The physicians at such estab-
lishments are most cruelly deceived by the patients.

A well conducted and properly managed hospital
—lunatic asylums are not necessary for the proper
carrying out of the cure—will offer all the necessary
guarantees for the successful conclusion of the treatment, and we must always bear in mind, with regard
to the latter, that although some cases may be
attended with no difficulty, it is impossible to decide

beforehand, whether the symptoms of the abstinence will be of a severe or a light nature.

I have remarked upon the different deceptions to which the medical attendant is exposed during the treatment of morbid craving for morphia, rendering it difficult and unsatisfactory. The absence of the symptoms of abstinence will, in many cases, soon convince the doctor that he is being deceived: the certainty of the deception, however, can only be proved by detecting morphia in the system.

I therefore took care to find a method by which it could be positively decided, within a short time, whether any morphia, and how much of it, had been taken by the patient.

The method of Professor Dragendorff[1] will satisfy all requirements even in case only a small quantity of urine is used. The qualitative analysis, which moreover may be made by every pharma ceutical chemist, can be finished within a period of four to five hours, the quantitative analysis taking eight to ten hours.

The mode of procedure is as follows: 100, respectively 50 cubic centimetres of urine are evaporated on the water-bath to a dry state, the residue is mixed with absolute alcohol, the insoluble salts are removed by filtration and the alcoholic filtrate is again evaporated. The residue is mixed with water,

---

[1] *Dragendorff*: 'Die gerichtlich-chemische Ermittelung von Giften.' Pctersburg, 1876 ; and *Levinstein*: 'Weitere Beiträge zur Pathologie der Morphiumsucht und der acuten Morphiumvergiftung.' Lecture delivered on Nov. 22, 1876.

again filtered, and, to remove the urea, is shaken with small quantities of amylic alcohol in a warm place, as long as it will take up colouring matter.

This amylic alcohol does not, as yet, contain morphia, but urea only.   It is, therefore, evaporated, and ammonia is added to the watery solution, so as to free the morphia contained therein from its combination with acid salts ; this alkaline watery solution is again shaken with amylic alcohol three or four times, and at last these four extracts are mixed, the amylic alcohol being removed by evaporation or distillation.

The residue contains the morphia, which may now be tested either by Fröhde's method (molybdenate of soda and sulphuric acid) or by the more reliable reaction of Husemann:[1] heating with concentrated sulphuric acid to 150° R. (302° F.), and then adding dilute nitric acid.

The morphia, with the exception of a very small quantity, passes away with the urine soon after its introduction into the system, and small doses of a-quarter of a grain have been traced with certainty (qualitatively) by the last-mentioned method.   In cases of morbid craving for morphia the evacuation is not very rapid, as the urine contains morphia for six to eight days after the commencement of the abstinence.   A patient, whose urine contains morphia for a longer period than six or eight days,

---

[1] Husemann : 'Die Pflanzenstoffe,' Berlin, 1871, p. 124.

is sure to be continuing the injections of morphia,
although he may himself positively deny the fact.

PROPHYLAXIS.

The successful study of prophylactic measures,
for the sake of preventing the further spreading of
morbid craving for morphia, is only to be carried on
by energetic mutual action on the part of the medical
practitioners, supported by the respective legal authorities. We shall not be wrong in saying that
morbid craving for morphia, after the lapse of several
years, will be of rare occurrence in Germany, as soon
as the governmental decrees, already issued by some
of the states, are obeyed ; the doctors in future not
allowing the morphia injections to be practised by
anyone but themselves.

On glancing over the different laws having reference thereto, I find a decree, dated September 27,
1725, prohibiting the chemists from making up prescriptions of unregistered medical men.

A medical decree of December 10, 1800, strictly
interdicts the sale of opium and its preparations to
the general public. Another decree of October 11,
1801, orders that prescriptions containing opium are
not to be repeated without the knowledge and renewed order of the respective physician.

In consequence of the alteration of the whole
legislation, relating to trade, the following decree
with reference to the sale of drugs and pharmaceutical preparations was published :—

'*Governmental Decree of March* 25, 1872, *relating to the Sale of Drugs and Pharmaceutical Preparations*—

'We, William, by the Grace of God Emperor of Germany, King of Prussia, etc., etc., decree in the name of the German Empire :

'SEC. 1. That the keeping for sale of all the preparations for curative purposes (morphia, etc.) enumerated in the subjoined Schedule A, is exclusively permitted to pharmaceutical chemists.

'SEC. 2. That the sale of all drugs and chemical preparations enumerated in the subjoined Schedule B (morphia, etc.) to the general public, is exclusively permitted to pharmaceutical chemists.

'In witness whereof our own signature and imperial great seal is affixed.

'WILLIAM, Imperator.

(L.S.)   'PRINCE VON BISMARCK.

'BERLIN :

'*March* 25, 1872.'

But experience showed that druggists, as well as pharmaceutical chemists, acted in defiance of the legal decrees, and that the latter, disregarding them, made up prescriptions of non-certified medical men.

To create a wider circle of legal enactments, the author on December 20, 1875, submitted a memorial with suggestions to the Royal Prussian Ministerial Department for clerical, educational, and medical affairs, containing principally the following regulations :—

1. The chemists are not allowed to dispense prescriptions ordering morphia, unless they are signed by a medical practitioner residing in the place, or pharmaceutical district, whose full name and address must be clearly written thereon.

In places where there are hundreds of medical

men, the pharmaceutical chemist is unable to examine into the correctness of all the signatures : he only knows that doctors of such names are residing in the place, but is not conversant with their hand-writing, and is unable to verify the signatures in doubtful cases. The case is different, however, if, besides his full name, the medical man writes his address on the prescription, because now the chemist is able to convince himself of the accuracy of the signature. Apart from rendering themselves liable to punishment, for falsifying a prescription, most persons will shrink from perpetrating an evident falsehood, while, on the other hand, they do not mind putting a well-known name under a morphia prescription, especially if that name does not desig-nate a special person.

2. Repetitions of prescriptions containing mor-phia are not allowed, every order for morphia requiring a new prescription, according to the rule given in 1.

The restrictions with regard to the prescriptions would relate to the dispensing of morphia for injec-tions, and not for the internal use of the drug. Together with the prohibition of the repetition, a decree would be found advisable, ordering the chemists to keep all the morphia prescriptions they have dispensed, for the purpose of official inspection at a later period.

3. The medical practitioners are to be called upon officially, to personally administer every injec-

tion, and not to leave this task to the patient, to his friends, to his assistants, to the midwife, the nurses, or the servants.

Up to the present time, however, no medical practitioner can, according to the present condition of the law, be compelled to do so : hence the personal administration of the injections is a demand upon the conscience of each individual medical man.

It is true that, at first, the doctor, especially in the country, will have to struggle with difficulties and opposition on the part of the patients, as he cannot at all times be with them ; and even material loss may be caused him through strictly doing his duty, but he will be rewarded by the knowledge of having averted harm from his patients which it is not easy to redress.

In consequence of this memorial, the following ministerial order, dated January 31, 1876, was issued :—

'*Ministerial Circular of January* 31, 1876, *addressed to all Royal Governmental Departments, Provincial Administrations, and the Royal President of Police, regarding the repetition of prescriptions for injections of morphia :*

'A complaint, on the part of the medical profession, has been lodged in my department, that chemists very frequently break the law with regard to the regulations issued on behalf of the dispensing and repetition of prescriptions, and especially that they not only repeat the prescriptions for injections of morphia, ordered by registered practitioners, without the latters' knowledge and consent, but that they also dispense the drug when prescribed by non-registered medical men. Considering the hurtful consequences that may arise out of such proceedings to the respective patients,

I take this opportunity to direct all Governmental Departments, etc., etc., to clearly point out to all pharmaceutical chemists in their respective districts the regulations prohibiting such a proceeding, as mentioned in the revised legal pharmaceutical enactments of October 11, 1801, as well as in the new decree of March 8, 1870, No. 641 M, and at the same time to order the medical officers of health to especially control the pharmaceutical chemists with regard to their acting in defiance of the above-mentioned legal decrees.

'Signed by Order,   SYDOW.

'Ministerial Department for Clerical
Educational, and Medical Affairs.

' BERLIN ·
' *January* 31, 1876. '

Notwithstanding this enactment, the chemists and druggists still dispense and sell morphia to the public in general.

There is, however, another way of preventing the spread of morbid craving for morphia, supporting at the same time the measures taken by the Government, and the position of the medical profession, *i.e.*, the public instruction by popular writings on the part of the official authorities, after the manner carried out by the Royal Prussian Government on several other occasions. Thus it annually publishes a warning in the Government organs, and the daily papers, regarding the use of poisonous colours and materials, and it annually repeats the instructions, in order to prevent intoxication by oxide of carbon, through using stoves with hermetically closing doors and without vent holes, etc., etc. In the same sense the Ministerial Department for Clerical,

Educational, and Medical Affairs ordered the police to instruct the public by official notifications as to the action of chloral.

No official instructions have, up to the present time, been published regarding the dangers attendant upon the abuse of injections of morphia. As soon, however, as the educated public, who is mostly afflicted with morbid craving for morphia, has acquired a knowledge of the great extent of the injury following the abuse of morphia, it will itself become, eventually, the guardian of its highest interests.

LONDON: PRINTED BY
SPOTTISWOODE AND CO, NEW-STREET SQUARE
AND PARLIAMENT STREET

SMITH, ELDER, & CO.'S PUBLICATIONS.

On the CONVOLUTIONS of the HUMAN BRAIN. By Dr. ALEX-
ANDER ECKER, Professor of Anatomy and Comparative Anatomy in the University of Freiburg,
Baden. Translated, by permission of the Author, by JOHN C. GALTON, M.A. Oxon., M.R.C.S.,
F.L.S. Post 8vo. 4s. 6d.

DEMONSTRATIONS of ANATOMY; being a Guide to the Know-
ledge of the Human Body by Dissection, By GEORGE VINER ELLIS, Professor of Anatomy in
University College, London. Seventh Edition, Revised. With 248 Engravings on Wood
Small 8vo. 12s. 6d. The number of illustrations has been largely added to in this edition, and
many of the new woodcuts are reduced copies of the Plates in the Author's work, 'Illustrations
of Dissections.'

ILLUSTRATIONS of DISSECTIONS. In a Series of Original
Coloured Plates, the Size of Life, representing the Dissection of the Human Body. By G. V.
ELLIS and G. H. FORD. Imperial folio, 2 vols. half-bound in morocco, £6. 6s. May also be
had in parts, separately. Parts 1 to 28, 3s. 6d. each ; Part 29, 5s.

On the PAST, PRESENT, and FUTURE of THERAPEUTICS.
Introductory to the Course of Materia Medica at St. Mary's Hospital. By ROBERT FARQUHARSON,
M.D. Edin., M.R.C.P.L., Lecturer on Materia Medica at St. Mary's Hospital Medical School. 1s.

The FUNCTIONS of the BRAIN. By DAVID FERRIER, M.D., F.R.S.,
Assistant-Physician to King's College Hospital ; Professor of Forensic Medicine, King's College.
With numerous Illustrations. 8vo. 15s.

The MAINTENANCE of HEALTH. A Medical Work for Lay
Readers. By J. MILNER FOTHERGILL, M.D., M.R.C.P., Assistant-Physician to the City of
London Hospital for Diseases of the Chest (Victoria Park), Physician to the West London
Hospital. Crown 8vo. 12s. 6d.

The PATHOLOGICAL ANATOMY of the NERVOUS CENTRES.
By EDWARD LONG FOX, M.D., F.R.C.S., F.R.C.P., Physician to the Bristol Royal Infirmary ;
late Lecturer on the Principles and Practice of Medicine and of Pathological Anatomy at the
Bristol Medical School. With Illustrations. 8vo. 12s. 6d.

OMPENDIUM of HISTOLOGY. Twenty-four Lectures. By HEIN-
RICH FREY, Professor. Translated from the German, by permission of the Author, by GEORGE
R. CUTTER, M.D. With 208 Illustrations, 8vo. 12s.

n the CONNECTION of BRIGHT'S DISEASE with CHANGES
in the VASCULAR SYSTEM. With Illustrations from the Sphymograph. By A. L. GALARIN,
M.A., M.D., Fellow of Trinity College, Cambridge. Demy 8vo. 1s. 6d.

USCULTATION and PERCUSSION, together with the other
Methods of Physical Examination of the Chest. By SAMUEL GEE, M.D. New Edition, with
Illustrations, fcp. 8vo. 5s. 6d.

SYSTEM of SURGERY : PATHOLOGICAL, DIAGNOSTIC,
THERAPEUTIC, and OPERATIVE. By SAMUEL D. GROSE, M.D., LL.D., D.C.L. Oxon.
Fifth Edition, greatly Enlarged and thoroughly revised, with upwards of 1,400 Illustrations.
2 vols. 8vo. £3. 10s.

PRACTICAL TREATISE on FRACTURES and DISLOCA
TIONS. By FRANK HASTINGS HAMILTON, A.M., M.D., LL.D. Fifth Edition, Revised and
Improved, with 322 Illustrations. 8vo. 28s.

MANUAL of PUBLIC HEALTH, for the Use of Local Authori-
ties, Medical Officers of Health, and others. By W. H. MICHAEL, F.C.S., Barrister-at-Law ;
W. H. CORFIELD, M.A., M.D. Oxon. ; and J. A. WANKLYN, M.R.C.S. Edited by ERNEST HART.
Post 8vo. 12s. 6d.

SSENTIALS of the PRINCIPLES and PRACTICE of MEDICINE.
A Handbook for Students and Practitioners. By HENRY HARTSHORNE, A.M., M.D. New
Edition. 12s. 6d.

he GEOGRAPHICAL DISTRIBUTION of HEART DISEASE
and DROPSY, CANCER in FEMALES, and PHTHISIS in FEMALES in ENGLAND and
WALES. Illustrated with six small and three large coloured Maps. By ALFRED HAVILAND,
Member of the Royal College of Surgeons, England, &c. &c. &c. Folio, 25s.

The ESSENTIALS of BANDAGING: including the Management of Fractures and Dislocations, with Directions for Using other Surgical Apparatus. With 128 Engravings. By BERKELEY HILL, M.B. Lond., F.R.C.S. Third Edition, Revised and Enlarged. Fcp. 8vo. 4s. 6d.

SYPHILIS and LOCAL CONTAGIOUS DISORDERS. By BERKELEY HILL, M.D. Lond., F.R.C.S. Demy 8vo. 16s.

SURGERY: its Principles and Practice. By TIMOTHY HOLMES, F.R.C.S. Surgeon to St. George's Hospital. With upwards of 400 Illustrations. Royal 8vo. 30s.

LECTURES on BRIGHT'S DISEASE, with Especial Reference to PATHOLOGY, DIAGNOSIS, and TREATMENT. By GEORGE JOHNSON, M.D., F.R.S., Fellow of the Royal College of Physicians, Physician to King's College Hospital, Professor of Medicine, King's College, &c. With numerous Illustrations. Post 8vo. 5s.

The ANATOMY of the LYMPHATIC SYSTEM. By E. KLEIN, M.D., F.R.S., Assistant Professor at the Laboratory of the Brown Institution, London, Lecturer on General Histology at the Medical School of St. Bartholomew's Hospital.

Part I. The Serous Membranes. With 10 Double-page Illustrations, 8vo. 10s. 6d.
Part II. The Lung. With Illustrations. 10s. 6d.

₊ These Researches are published with the sanction and approval of the Medical Officer of the Privy Council. The Government Grant Committee of the Royal Society have furnished means for the execution of the Plates.

A HANDBOOK of OPHTHALMIC SURGERY. By BENJAMIN THOMPSON LOWNE, F.R.C.S., Ophthalmic Surgeon to the Great Northern Hospital. Crown 8vo. 6s.

HANDBOOK of RURAL SANITARY SCIENCE. Illustrating the best means of securing Health and preventing Disease. Edited by LORY MARSH, M.D., Member of the Royal College of Physicians, London; Member of the Royal College of Surgeons, England. Crown 8vo. 6s.

INJURIES of NERVES and their CONSEQUENCES. By By S. WEIR MITCHELL, M.D. 8vo. 15s.

NOTES of DEMONSTRATIONS of PHYSIOLOGICAL CHEMIS- TRY. By S. W. MOORE, Junior Demonstrator of Practical Physiology at St. George's Medical School, Fellow of the Chemical Society, &c. Crown 8vo. 3s. 6d.

On FUNCTIONAL DERANGEMENTS of the LIVER. By C. MURCHISON. M.D., LL.D., F.R.S., Physician and Lecturer on Medicine, St. Thomas's Hospital, and formerly on the Medical Staff of H.M.'s Bengal Army. Crown 8vo. 5s.

The EXAMINER in ANATOMY: A Course of Instruction on the Method of Answering Anatomical Questions. By ARTHUR TREHERN NORTON, F.R.C.S., Assistant-Surgeon, Surgeon in Charge of the Throat Department, Lecturer on Surgery, and late Lecturer on Anatomy at St. Mary's Hospital, &c. &c. 8vo. 5s.

A PRACTICAL and THEORETICAL TREATISE on DISEASES of the SKIN. By GEORGE NAYLOR, F.R.C.S. Second Edition, with Illustrations. 8vo. 12s. 6d.

A GUIDE to URINARY ANALYSIS, for the Use of Physicians and Students. By HENRY G. PIFFARD, A.M., M.D. Demy 8vo. 7s. 6d.

A TREATISE on the SCIENCE and PRACTICE of MIDWIFERY. By W. S. PLAYFAIR, M.D., F.R.C.P., Professor of Obstetric Medicine in King's College; Physician for the Diseases of Women and Children to King's College Hospital; Examiner in Midwifery to the University of London, and lately to the Royal College of Physicians; Vice- President of the Obstetrical Society, &c. With 166 Illustrations. 2 vols. 8vo. 28s.

London: SMITH, ELDER, & CO., 15 Waterloo Place.

A TEXT-BOOK of ELECTRICITY in MEDICINE and SURGERY,
for the Use of Students and Practitioners. By GEORGE VIVIAN POORE, M.D. Lond., M.R.C.P.,
&c., Assistant-Physician to University College Hospital ; Senior Physician to the Royal Infirmary
for Children and Women. Crown 8vo. 8s. 6d.

QUAIN and WILSON'S ANATOMICAL PLATES. 201 Plates.
2 vols. Royal folio, half-bound in morocco, or 5 Parts bound in cloth. Price, coloured,
£10. 10s.; plain £6. 6s.

A MANUAL of TOXICOLOGY, including the Consideration of the
Nature, Properties, Effects, and Means of Detection of Poisons, more especially in their
Medico-Legal Relations. By JOHN J. REESE, M.D. 8vo. 12s. 6d.

A PRACTICAL TREATISE on URINARY and RENAL
DISEASES, including URINARY DEPOSITS. Illustrated by numerous Cases and Engravings.
By WILLIAM ROBERTS, M.D. Third Edition, revised and enlarged. Small 8vo. 12s. 6d.

246 Outline Drawings with adhesive backs, for Clinical Case Books.

OUTLINE DIAGRAM FORMS for CLINICAL CASE BOOKS.
For the representation of Injuries and Diseases and Physical Signs. Designed for the use of
Clinical Students, Physicians and Surgeons. By G. ROWELL, M.D., Resident Surgeon to the
Leeds Infirmary. 3s. 6d.

SPINAL DISEASE and SPINAL CURVATURE : their Treatment
by Suspension and the Use of Plaster-of-Paris Bandage. By LEWIS A. SAYRE, M.D., of New
York, Professor of Orthopædic Surgery in Bellevue Hospital Medical College, New York,
&c. &c. Large crown 8vo. with 21 Photographs and numerous Woodcuts, 10s. 6d.

A COURSE of PRACTICAL HISTOLOGY. By EDWARD ALBERT
SCHÄFER, Assistant-Professor of Physiology, University College. With numerous Illustrations.
Crown 8vo. 10s. 6d.

COMMENTARY on the BRITISH PHARMACOPŒIA. By WALTER
GEORGE SMITH, M.D., Fellow and Censor, King and Queen's College of Physicians [in Ireland ;
Examiner in Materia Medica, Q.U.I. ; Assistant-Physician to the Adelaide Hospital. Crown
8vo. 12s. 6d.

An EPITOME of THERAPEUTICS. Being a Comprehensive Sum-
mary of the Treatment of Disease as recommended by the leading British, American, and
Continental Physicians. By W. DOMETT STONE, M.D., F.R.C.S. Crown 8vo. 8s. 6d.

An INTRODUCTION to the STUDY of CLINICAL MEDICINE :
being a Guide to the Investigation of Disease, for the Use of Students. By OCTAVIUS STURGES,
M.D. Cantab., F.R.C.P., Physician to Westminster Hospital. Crown 8vo. 4s. 6d.

The NATURAL HISTORY and RELATIONS of PNEUMONIA :
a Clinical Study. By OCTAVIUS STURGES, M.D., F.R.C.P., Physician to the Westminster
Hospital. Crown 8vo. 10s. 6d.

A PRACTICAL TREATISE on the DISEASES of the HEART
and GREAT VESSELS ; including the Principles of their Physical Diagnosis. By WALTER
HAYLE WALSHE, M.D. Fourth Edition, thoroughly revised and greatly enlarged. Demy
8vo. 16s.

A PRACTICAL TREATISE on DISEASES of the LUNGS :
including the Principles of Physical Diagnosis, and Notes on Climate. By WALTER HAYLE
WALSHE, M.D. Fourth Edition, revised and much enlarged. Demy 8vo. 16s.

MANUAL of LUNACY : a Handbook relating to the Legal Care and
Treatment of the Insane in the Public and Private Asylums of Great Britain, Ireland, United
States of America, and the Continent. By LYTTLETON S. FORBES WINSLOW, M.B. and M.L.
Cantab.; M.R.C.P. Lond.; D.C.L. Oxon. With a Preface by FORBES WINSLOW, M.D.
Post 8vo. 12s. 6d.

A TREATISE on THERAPEUTICS : comprising Materia Medica
and Toxicology, with especial reference to the Application of the Physiological Action
of Drugs to Clinical Medicine. By H. C. WOOD, Jun., M.D. 8vo. New Edition. 14s.

London : SMITH, ELDER, & CO., 15 Waterloo Place.

CPSIA information can be obtained
at www.ICGtesting.com
Printed in the USA
LVOW04s0416090216
474198LV00031BA/1239/P